What Shall I Do About My Death?

Advance Planning: A Guide to Writing an *Advance Decision* & a *Statement of Values*,

Plus All you need to know about death and dying, and *Do Not Attempt to Resuscitate* agreements

Dr. Hilary Page

This book was set in *Adobe InDesign CS3* by John P. Frisby.

Printed and bound by Lightning Source.

Published by Mospeate Publishing, Mospeate House, Sheffield S10 3RG.

ISBN 978_0_9564949_3_1 (pbk)

Family Relationships: Death and Bereavement; Elder Law; Home and Community Care.

For Our Parents

Acknowledgements
I am indebted to colleagues, friends and family for help, advice and
encouragement, and especially to my husband for his calm and
cheerful support. Thank you.

Thank you to everyone who talked with me about their experiences
of witnessing death and their hopes for themselves
when the time comes.

Thank you to the doctors and nurses and others who looked after
our parents at their deaths.

First published by Mospeate Publishing October 2010
Second Edition October 2015

CONTENTS

PREFACE   *i-ix*

CHAPTER 1 WHAT SHALL I DO ABOUT MY DEATH?   1-12
A good death? Dying; life-sustaining treatment. The Advance Decision; Mental Capacity Act. Do Not Attempt to Resuscitate. Care Pathways; Report of the National Audit Office; NHS End of Life Care Strategy. Advance Planning. Choices for your family after your death. The debate about assisted suicide.

CHAPTER 2 DYING   13-34
What do people die from? Vital functions. The need for water and food. Making the right decision about artificial feeding. Progress and trajectories of chronic disease: respiratory disease; heart disease; stroke; cancer; dementia; dying from old age. Palliative Care. What are the last days like? Local Care Pathways .

CHAPTER 3 LIFE-SUSTAINING TREATMENTS   35-54
What are life-sustaining treatments? Life-sustaining treatment and palliative care; artificial hydration and nutrition; pacemakers; antibiotics; blood transfusion; renal dialysis. Treatments for respiratory failure: oxygen by mask; ventilation. Switching off the ventilator. Life-sustaining operations.

CHAPTER 4 WRITING YOUR ADVANCE DECISION TO REFUSE TREATMENT   55-100
Living wills. Statement of Values; The *Mental Capacity Act*; loss of mental capacity; communication difficulties. Why write an *Advance Decision?* How to write an *Advance Decision*. Example of an *Advance Decision*. Detailed instructions. Useful websites. Lasting Power of Attorney.

CHAPTER 5 DO NOT ATTEMPT TO RESUSCITATE   101-110
Cardiopulmonary resuscitation (CPR); cardiac defibrillation; the chance of successful resuscitation? The *Do Not Attempt to Resuscitate* (DNAR) agreement. DNAR and detailed instructions

in an *Advance Decision*. Deciding to withdraw life-sustaining treatment. Policy in terminal care settings: giving patients the opportunity to decide; training for doctors and nurses; DNAR at home.

CHAPTER 6 THE CHOICE OF WHERE TO DIE   *111-136*
Dying: in your own home; in a care home; in hospital. Dying in a hospice. How does the trajectory of disease affect the place of death? Advance Planning: make staying at home feasible. Preferred place of death. How a *Statement of Values* can help. The role of the Advance Decision and the Statement of Values. An example of a Statement of Values.

CHAPTER 7 DECISIONS ABOUT YOUR BODY   *137-150*
AFTER DEATH
Plan your funeral ceremony. Cremation or burial? Post-mortem examination. NHS Organ Donor Register. Donating your brain for research. Donating your body.

CHAPTER 8 WHAT SHALL I DO NOW?   *151-156*
Write an Advance Decision and a Statement of Values: discuss these with your family. If you hope to die at home, plan in advance. Register with the NHS Organ Donor Registry. For financial affairs, grant the Power of Attorney. Be informed about the role of the DNAR agreement, and the current debate about assisted suicide.

APPENDIX BLANK FORM FOR ADVANCE DECISION   *157-168*

INDEX   *169*

PREFACE

Preliminary remarks: I emphasise that this book is not about assisted dying (called by some assisted suicide). The debate on that has been vigorous in recent years. However, the rejection by a large majority of the House of Commons in 2015 of a bill to permit assisted dying in certain circumstances means that there is little prospect of any change of the law for the foreseeable future.

I do not express my personal view on that debate in this book. Rather, my intention is to explain what can be done legally at the present time in controlling the circumstances of one's death. That is, to write an Advance Decision .

Any mentally competent adult has the legal right to give informed consent, or to refuse medical treatment. The Advance Decision is a means of carrying this right forward to a situation in the future when a person has lost mental capacity.

By writing an Advance Decision now, while of sound mind, you can refuse life sustaining treatment, in future circumstances where you are terminally ill and have lost mental capacity. You can be allowed to die, if possible in your home, with care aimed at making you comfortable, instead of having invasive efforts made to keep you alive.

My father wrote an Advance Decision. He got the form through the post, filled it in, and wrote a letter to his family saying it was our moral duty to follow his wishes. When he lost mental capacity, after his third stroke, we showed his Advance Decision to the doctor looking after him. From then on the family were involved in discussions about his illness: What exactly had happened to him? Had he really lost Mental Capacity? What outcome could be expected from treatment? To what extent might there be any recovery? Together we considered what would be his wishes about medical treatment.

We felt empowered because of what he had said to us and written in his Advance Decision. He was allowed to die, with excellent care, and not kept alive in a state he would have hated by medical treatment which would have been invasive.

I decided to write an Advance Decision for myself. I looked on the Internet for a form to download and fill in. There are plenty of forms, all good in parts. However, the general advice was to discuss it with my doctor, and there was an underlying assumption that I already had a fatal or progressive disease. I found the Advance Decision had been taken up into the realms of professionals - particularly cancer care specialists and specialists in palliative care. The envisaged scenario was that people would be prompted and guided by their doctor in the writing of an Advance Decision, when they had reached an advanced stage of terminal illness, typically cancer, or after an early diagnosis of dementia (though it must be done while you are still mentally capable).

It was not expected that a healthy individual (like me) should take it into their head to write an Advance Decision. I decided to write this book, to encourage people to think and talk about death, and to write an Advance Decision themselves, while they are well.

The legal status of an Advance Decision to refuse life prolonging treatment is ratified by the Mental Capacity Act. Legal aspects are important if there is a dispute, but this would be rare. Doctors welcome guidance with the difficult and sensitive decisions they have to make, when someone is terminally ill, but unable to speak for themselves.

Doctors are interested in a person's motivation to write an Advance Decision, and the discussions with their family or close friends about what their wishes and fears would be, if in future they might be terminally ill and have lost mental capacity.

In a Statement of Values you describe your motivation and the background to your Advance Decision

Although relevant to many more people than the proposals on assisted dying, the Advance Decision is ignored by the media. I hope there will be a change in the way the Advance Decision is presented, to encourage every capable adult to write one. No one knows when accident or illness may deprive them of mental capacity. Professional advice is not needed, but it will be helpful to people to have a suitable form.

My own Advance Decision is included as an example, and there is a spare form at the back of the book, and at my website advancedecision.co.uk. I have incorporated in the form, (with reference and acknowledgement) some good ideas which I discovered in my research for this book.

Hilary Page   October 2015

The meaning of the word 'Family'

Throughout this book I have referred to 'family' in the context of discussions about an Advance Decision.

Please take this word 'family' to have a wide application. It includes parents, offspring and siblings, marriage partners and civil partners. However many people are closer to workmates, friends, partners, neighbours or to their carers.

It is difficult to cover these possibilities without being long winded, so I have used the word 'family' as shorthand.

Chapter 1
What Shall I Do About My Death?

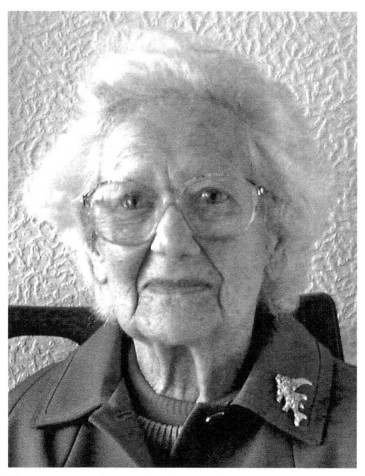

They are not long, the days of wine and roses:
Out of a misty dream
Our path emerges for a while, then closes.
                    Ernest Dowson (1867-1900).

A newspaper columnist, Polly Toynbee, wrote from personal experience of a death in her family, describing 'a conspiracy of silence about the actual processes of death'.[2] I decided to break that silence with the first edition of this book. I have tried to encapsulate what I know about death as a doctor and a daughter, and what I learned while writing my own Advance Decision and Statement of Values.

The Advance Decision enables you, in advance, while you are mentally capable, to refuse life sustaining treatment if at some time in the future you have a terminal illness, and have lost the mental capacity to take part in decisions about your medical care. It is a plea for palliative care, (see p. 31) to allow you to die peacefully, if possible at home. Your Statement of Values (see pp. 75, 129) explains the motivation for your Advance Decision and describes situations which you would find intolerable. This Statement can also indicate your wishes for personal aspects of care, and for your body after death. This book will stimulate discussion with your family about death and dying. These discussions, and the legal status of your Advance Decision will empower your family to initiate open and honest discussion with your doctors and nurses, so that treatment will be in accordance with your wishes.

Is There Such a Thing as a Good Death?

A discussion group convened by *Age Concern* outlined twelve *Principles of a Good Death.*[3] I have summarised the first eleven as:

Principles of a Good Death – Age Concern

Know when death is coming and understand what to expect.

Retain control of what happens.

Enjoy privacy and dignity.

Be in control of the relief of pain and other symptoms.

Choose where to die.

Have access to information and expertise.

Receive emotional and spiritual support.

Have access to hospice care.

Choose who may visit you and who shares the end.

Have time to say goodbye.

Choose not to have life pointlessly prolonged.

These first eleven principles apply to a person who remains mentally capable, aware of what is happening to them and also able to express their wishes and take part in decisions about their care.

Many dying people lose mental capacity, some shortly before the end, others through dementia of long duration. Writing an Advance Decision gives you the opportunity to influence your death even if you lose mental capacity.

Therefore the twelfth and last principle from Age Concern is:

Be able to write a living will and be confident your wishes will be respected.

I was influenced by the deaths of my parents. My mother died from Alzheimers. She had often spoken to us about an Advance Directive, but never got round to writing one. In the late stages of her disease life prolonging treatment was proposed which we were sure she would not have wanted. My father persuaded the doctors that she would have found it hateful to live on without her mind, unable to walk, incontinent and needing to be artificially fed.

After she died, my father wrote his Advance Directive, (now known as an Advance Decision[4]). Later, after his third stroke, it was apparent he would not recover mental capacity. He was allowed to die peacefully, with palliative care, rather than being kept alive by life sustaining treatment. His Advance Directive made clear what he wanted.

Dying and Life-sustaining Treatment

I hope to demystify the natural processes of dying, and explain the medical treatments which can be used to keep a person alive. Knowing more about these will motivate you to write your own *Advance Decision* and Statement of Values.

The Mental Capacity Act 2005[4]

The mental Capacity Act of 2005 came into effect in October 2007 introducing the new legal status of the *Advance Decision to Refuse Treatment*. The Advance Decision can allow you to refuse life sustaining treatment in circumstances where you would prefer to be allowed to die, but are unable through loss of mental capacity, to direct your medical treatment.

Chapter Four is about the *Advance Decision to Refuse Treatment* and other provisions of the Mental Capacity Act. (In Scotland, the Adults with Incapacity Act [Scotland] 2000). My own Advance Decision is at the end of Chapter Four, and there is a spare form at the back of the book.

This book will help you decide whether to appoint a *welfare attorney* to make health decisions for you if you lose mental capacity. For most people it will not be necessary to appoint a welfare attorney, although an attorney to look after your financial affairs may be important. (See pp.91-94.)

General Medical Council Guidance for Doctors[5]

'Guidance on treatment and care at the end of life' was issued in 2010. This is applicable across the UK. (See pp. 57, 87, 89.)

Joint Statement on Cardiopulmonary Resuscitation[6]

The Royal College of Nursing and the Royal College of Physicians have produced a *Joint Statement on Cardiopulmonary Resuscitation* (CPR). In some circumstances resuscitation would not be welcome or appropriate. Advance planning and discussion with the patient, (or with the family or representative if the patient is not mentally capable), may lead to a *Do Not Attempt to Resuscitate* (DNAR) agreement. The joint statement considers in depth the medical and ethical issues and the need for training of doctors and nurses who will be involved in decisions about resuscitation. The DNAR agreement is discussed in Chapter Five.

Report of the National Audit Office on End of Life Care[7]
In November 2008 the National Audit Office reported on the services provided for dying people. In general people do not die where they want to. The National Audit Office found that most people wish to be cared for and die in their homes.

Of the half million people who die each year in England, the majority die in hospital. A detailed study of patients' records in one Primary Care Trust revealed that 40% of those who died in hospital did not have a medical need to be there, and nearly one quarter of these had been in hospital for over a month.

The findings of the National Audit Office put pressure on National and Local Government, the NHS and Social Services to unify their approach to the care of dying people in the community and shift the emphasis away from hospitals.

Change is In the Air!
In the current climate of austerity and change, government and professionals want to consolidate the care of dying people, across NHS and Social Care budgets. More people will be enabled to die at home, supported by NHS community nurses and means tested agency based carers. People will be more in control if they think about dying, talk about it with their family and friends and write an Advance Decision supported by a Statement of Values.

In dying the main barrier to better care is that doctors and nurses find it difficult to open discussion about death. A recent poll by the Dying Matters Coalition[8] showed that members of the public are not keen to broach the subject of death with either their GP or their family. 'A mere 7% had discussed what sort of care they would want if they were unable to make their own decisions'. Around a third of GPs in the UK do not talk to older patients approaching death about their wishes. Clearly it will help if more people take the initiative in saying clearly what they want, in an Advance Decision.

An Advance Decision helps your family to open discussion about the possibility of your death. In clinical circumstances which you describe, if you have lost mental capacity, it enables doctors and nurses looking after you to provide care aimed at your comfort and dignity, recognising by your Advance Decision your legal right to refuse consent to life sustaining treatment.

The NHS End of Life Care Strategy[9]

The NHS End of Life Care Strategy was published in July 2008, promoting high quality care for **all** adults at the end of life, not only those dying from cancer, which has been the focus of palliative care for so long.

Key points are that people should have more choice about where they want to live and die, and that care should be provided in peoples' homes and in care homes in the community as far as possible.

Gold Standards Framework for Community Palliative Care[10]

Palliative care is the holistic care of patients with advanced, progressive, incurable illness, focused on the management of a patient's pain and other distressing symptoms, and the provision of psychological, social and spiritual support to patients and their families. Palliative care is not dependent on diagnosis or prognosis, and can be provided at any at any stage of a patient's illness, not only in the last few days of life. The objective is to support patients to live as well as possible until they die and to die with dignity[5](see p. 31).

The Royal College of General Practitioners has agreed the standards for care which service providers should aim for and measure themselves against. The existence of agreed standards will help improve the services to people dying in their own homes or in care homes in the community. The Framework includes examples of good practice which have been developed in different places, and recommends that these approaches should be more widely used. They recognise that *the greatest difficulty is acknowledging that the patient is dying*, and the framework therefore puts great emphasis on training doctors, nurses and others to feel comfortable raising issues of concern to people approaching death, and their families.

Advance Planning and Preferred Priorities for Care[11]

Advance Planning depends on thinking about death and discussing your wishes with your family and writing an Advance Decision. When someone is terminally ill and death is accepted, *Advance Planning* will be based on their *Preferred Priorities for Care*.

This will enable more people who wish it to die peacefully in their own home or in a care home close to where their friends and family live. Those providing care find out what aspects of care are most important to the patient and their family. They agree with the patient and the family how they will respond when there is a sudden worsening of the patient's condition, which otherwise might result in emergency admission to hospital, or other decisions being taken hurriedly, contrary to the patient's wishes. The factors which influence where people die are discussed in Chapter Six.

Pathways of Care for the Dying Patient

A Palliative Care Pathway was developed by *Marie Curie Cancer Care,* initially for cancer patients. With the help of doctors and

7

nurses at Liverpool University it was extended for people dying from any terminal illness - The Liverpool Care Pathway.[12]

The *Pathway* was controversial[13].People complained that it had been started without the consent of the patient or discussion with family members, and that dying patients had been 'deprived of fluids and food'. The *Liverpool Care Pathway* was reviewed by the *Department of Health* and later withdrawn.

A survey of Palliative Medicine Consultants[14] showed that 89% believe the Liverpool Care Pathway represents best practice for the care of dying patients and would choose it for themselves. The survey showed no barrier to eating, drinking or taking antibiotics and fluids while on the pathway if appropriate for symptom management. 'This survey gives overwhelming support for the Liverpool Care Pathway from doctors who have experience of caring for patients in the last few days of life.' Structured systems of care continue to be used but now take more account of local arrangements, which vary from one type of locality to another.

NICE Guidance for End of Life Care for Adults

The National Institute for Health and Care Excellence (see p. 127) has published Guidance consolidating the initiatives described in this chapter[15], and providing standards for evelution and regulation of Health and Social Services by the Care Quality Commission.[16]

Help Your Family After Your Death

There are choices for disposal of the body and funeral ceremonies, and there are medico-legal matters to consider, such as post mortem examination, organ donation and donation of your body. Chapter Seven is about these choices, including my own choices.

Assisted Dying

Lord Joffe's Bill on *Assisted Dying* presented to Parliament in 2004 proposed to legalise a doctor prescribing a fatal drug for someone terminally ill who wishes to die, and others assisting them to end their life by taking the drug.[17]It was defeated but assisted dying remains on the political agenda. The Parliamentary Group on Choice at the End of Life presented a consultation document: 'Safeguarding Choice'[18] in November 2012, and a new Bill on Assisted Dying[19] was brought to the House of Lords by Lord Falconer, in 2014. It was due for its second reading in the House of Lords but ran out of time before the general election of 2015. It was revived as a private members Bill by the Labour MP Bob Marris[20], but rejected by a vote of 330 to 118 at its second reading in the House of Commons in September 2015.[21]

People who are in unbearable circumstances, or fear they will be in the near future, because of an illness they have, will seek assisted suicide. They will arouse public sympathy and stimulate ongoing debate about this controversial issue.

In writing your Advance Decision to Refuse Treatment you are not indicating that you would be either for or against the legalisation of Assisted Dying.

Assisted Dying would involve someone helping a mentally capable person to die, at their own request, who is terminally ill and expected to die within six months. They must show a voluntary, clear and settled wish to end their life, and themselves take the final action of swallowing the lethal drug. Natural death would not have occurred at this time. This is assisted suicide, (although the term assisted dying seems more acceptable).[22]

An Advance Decision comes into effect if someone has lost mental capacity and is dying. By their Advance Decision they refuse to give consent for treatment aimed solely at sustaining their life, and can be allowed to die a natural death.

REFERENCES

1. Ernest Dowson (1867-1900). *Life's short span forbids us to enter on far-reaching hopes.* (Quotation from Horace.) In: *New Oxford Book of English Verse.* Ed. Helen Gardner. Oxford University Press 1974.

2. Toynbee P. *The Myth of Dying.* The Guardian. 25th March 2005.

3. *The future of health and care for older people: the best is yet to come.* The Millennium Papers: Debate of the Age. *Age Concern* 1999.

4. *The Mental Capacity Act.* Office of Public Sector Information (Legislation). The National Archives 2005.

5. *Treatment and care towards the end of life: good practice in decision making.* Guidance for doctors. General Medical Council 2010.

6. *Decisions Relating to Cardiopulmonary Resuscitation.* British Medical Association, Resuscitation Council UK and the Royal College of Nursing. BMA Publications 2007.

7. *End of Life Care.* National Audit Office. Stationery Office 2008.

8. *Millions leave it too late to discuss dying wishes.* Com Res survey commissioned by Dying Matters Coalition. National Council for Palliative Care May 2014.

9. *End of Life Care Strategy: Promoting high quality care for all adults at the end of life.* Department of Health 2008.

10. *A Programme for Community Palliative Care.* The Royal College of General Practitioners and the Gold Standards Framework (GSF) Central Team. NHS End of Life Care Programme. RCGP Publications 2008.

11. *Preferred Priorities for Care (PPC) NHS End of Life Care Programme.* Lancashire and South Cumbria Cancer Services Network and the National PPC Review Team. NHS End of Life Care Programme 2007.

12. *The Liverpool Primary Care Pathway for the Dying Patient. Version 11.* NHS End of Life Care Programme. Marie Curie Institute of Palliative Care. The University of Liverpool 2009.

13. Heidi Blake. *'All I ask is to die with dignity' Doctors hope that new guidelines on the Liverpool Care Pathway will allay families' fears.* The Daily Telegraph November 23rd 2009.

14. Krishna Chinthapalli. *Nine out of ten palliative care experts would choose the Liverpool Care Pathway.* British Medical Journal; 346: 2-3. 2013.

15. Guidance for End of Life Care for Adults. National Institute for Health and Care Excellence. NICE Quality standard [QS13] Published 2011 revised 2013.Website nice.org.uk

16. Care Quality Commission. The independent regulator of health and social care in England. Website cqg.org.uk 2015.

17. Lord Joel Joffe. *The Assisted Dying for the Terminally Ill Bill.* The House of Lords 2004.

18. All Party Parliamentary Group on Choice at the End of Life. *Safeguarding Choice. A Draft Assisted Dying Bill for Consultation.* The Houses of Parliament 2012.

19. *Assisted Dying Bill.* Private Members Bill sponsored by Lord Falconer of Thornton (HL) 2013-14. Website parliament.uk January 2014.

20. *Bill on Assisted Dying Bill.* Private Members Bill sponsored by Bob Marris and Lord Falconer of Thornton. Website parliament.uk September 2015.

21. MPs reject Assisted Dying Bill by two to one. The Times. 12 September, 2015.

22. Pratchett, T. *The 2010 Richard Dimbleby Lecture: Shaking Hands with Death.* Published in Pratchett, T. *A Slip of the Keyboard.* 2014. Transworld Publishers: London. pp.333-355.

Chapter 2
Dying

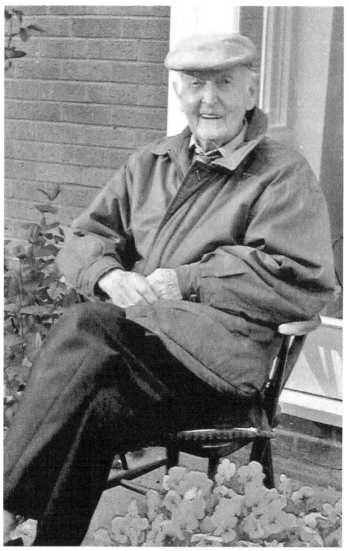

O teach me to see Death and not to fear,
But rather to take truce!   *Henry King (1592-1669)*

This chapter has been based on the acceptance that death can and will occur. The body will stop functioning. No more movement, no more eating, drinking, no more breathing, no more beating heart, no more seeing, hearing, tasting, touching, thinking.

Sudden unexpected death in the midst of life is not necessarily a good death, it is untimely and the raw grief of the family in these circumstances is terrible. However, people often say 'that's the way to go', especially if the person has had 'a good innings' and 'is lucky enough to die in their sleep'. Sometimes sudden death can intervene in the longer course of a disease, and this, depending on how far advanced that disease is, may sometimes be regarded as a release.

Most lives end in a slower process and there is choice about how the end of life is approached. This chapter is about what happens as the body dies – how the systems of the body can fail and life be stilled. Just as death can be shocking, some of the contents of this chapter are shocking. But I don't apologise – you can see worse things than I describe on the television every day of the week. It's called 'entertainment'. So don't be squeamish – look death squarely in the face. It will help you decide about an **Advance Decision.**

What Do People Die From?

Cancer, heart disease, respiratory disease and stroke are the four most frequent causes of death, with cancer predominating in the younger age groups (see Table 1). Dementia is a disease of old age, a major cause of death among the very elderly, and particularly pertinent to this book because of the loss of mental capacity involved.

The cause of death affects the choices that can be made about the place of death and the arrangements for care. Cancer patients

Table 1 Causes of Death (ONS 2015)[2]

Rates per million men and women in each age group

Cause of death	Cancer	Dementia	Heart Disease	Stroke	Respiratory Disaease
Age group M/F					
45-54 M	907	5	656	113	170
F	1053	6	172	89	126
55-64 M	3380	50	1774	287	646
F	2863	46	531	193	468
65-74 M	8682	346	4148	923	2274
F	6114	323	1744	701	1597
75-84 M	18367	3171	11679	3727	8083
F	11642	3553	7173	3545	5706
85+ M	33383	16091	33868	13241	29987
F	18951	21648	26428	14544	22367

are more likely than others to die at home or in a hospice; most deaths from dementia occur in nursing homes or care homes; most deaths from stroke, heart disease or respiratory disease occur in hospital.

The Audit Commission[3] drew attention to the disparity between people's preference for death at home or in a care home, and the fact that most people die in hospital. Reasons for this include lack of help in the community, people living alone, and the difficulty of knowing and accepting (for professionals as well as carers and family) that someone is actually dying. They recognised that even when planning for death at home, hospital admission may be needed to help with distressing symptoms particularly when someone is dying from heart or respiratory disease.

The choice of where to die will depend on many factors and is discussed in more detail in Chapter 6.

BEING ALIVE: VITAL FUNCTIONS

The vital functions which maintain life from moment to moment are:

The beating of the heart

The circulation of the blood

Breathing

These functions happen unconsciously and are driven from lower part of the brain, called the brain stem. So the fourth vital function is:

Activity of the brain stem

WHEN VITAL FUNCTIONS CEASE

The Heartbeat

If the heart stops beating, as in a heart attack, death occurs after three to four minutes.

The Circulation

The circulation stops if the heart stops. The effective circulation of the blood will fail if there is severe bleeding. The time taken to die will depend on how quickly blood is lost.

The Breathing

If breathing stops or is obstructed, death occurs in about five minutes.

The Brain Stem

The brain stem can be suddenly damaged by injury or stroke. More usually during the process of dying, the brain stem is starved of oxygen as the breathing, heartbeat and circulation gradually fail. The brain stem may be poisoned by substances which build up in the blood stream because other organs such as the kidneys or the liver are not working properly. At a critical point, the brain stem will cease to provide an adequate stimulus to maintain breathing or the heartbeat and death will follow.

SUDDEN DEATH IN TERMINAL ILLNESS
Not everyone dying from terminal illness fades gradually right to the end. Terminally ill people can die suddenly from a heart attack, or a massive stroke which damages the brain stem. This is more likely if there has been a previous heart attack or stroke. Sudden death may also occur during a chest infection, particularly in a person who has severe respiratory disease or heart failure.

Sudden death can occur from a pulmonary embolism. When the circulation is sluggish and the blood is thickened due to dehydration or other causes, there is a risk of a blood clot forming in the main vein of the leg - a deep vein thrombosis (DVT). The leg swells and is painful; a fragment of the clot can break off and be carried in the bloodstream to the heart and into the lung – a pulmonary embolus. The damage to the lung may be immediately fatal.

Vomiting may cause sudden death if the vomit is inhaled into the lungs. This can happen when the cough reflex is damaged due to a stroke, neurological degeneration, dementia or diminished consciousness.

Sudden death can also occur if cancer erodes into a blood vessel, causing massive haemorrhage. The bleeding is usually internal and therefore not visible, but it is painful. It is horrible if bleeding is external, perhaps from the lungs, stomach or bowel.

MORE GRADUAL DYING
The body does not usually die from the sudden catastrophic

failure of one system. Because all the organs of the body are interdependent, in ageing or in terminal illness everything runs down together. There is a knock-on effect as the whole body is failing and each problem causes something else to go wrong. Contrast this with a resilient and healthy young person whose body responds more successfully to illness because most organs of the body are working well except for the damaged part.

Inability to maintain sufficient fluid intake, and poor nourishment, are usual in the last days of life.

Water – a Vital Necessity

A dying person may be unable to swallow. Stroke, neurological degeneration or dementia can interrupt the swallowing reflex so the person chokes even on a sip of water. Injury or cancer can damage the mouth, throat or oesophagus (gullet) and make drinking impossible. Terminally ill people seem to lose their ability to feel thirsty - they forget to drink and gradually become dehydrated. Carers can prompt or help them to drink but it becomes more difficult to persuade them.

With dehydration the body loses its ability to maintain the internal environment. Toxic substances become concentrated and are not metabolised fast enough by the liver or excreted fast enough by the kidneys. Renal failure can develop if there is insufficient fluid to allow the kidneys to work properly. The disturbance of the body's internal environment means the vital organs begin to fail - the brain, heart and lungs. The circulation becomes sluggish so the supply of oxygen around the body is poor and the reduced flow of urine may lead to urinary infection which can further damage the kidneys and may be fatal.

Fluid can be provided by a 'drip', but even with a drip most people when they die are dehydrated to some degree. In any case their heart and kidneys could not cope with the amount of fluid required for normal hydration.

Food – Vital Nutrition

Lack of nutrition is not an immediate cause of death. Energy not obtained from food is instead obtained from the body fat and muscle. This abnormal metabolism produces toxins which build up and damage the vital organs. Because of lack of iron and other nutrients, the blood becomes less capable of supplying oxygen. Death from lack of food comes when the vital organs fail.

The organs which suffer most as the breathing, heartbeat and circulation become less efficient are those most demanding of oxygen - the brain, heart and kidneys. The heart deprived of oxygen becomes weaker and unstable. As the kidneys fail, fluid balance becomes precarious. Products of the abnormal metabolism which would normally be detoxified by the liver and excreted by the kidneys are retained and cause further damage. Such 'poisoning' building up gradually over a few weeks, and the chronic lack of oxygen in the blood, may cause the heart to falter and then to stop; it may depress breathing or interfere with the function of the brain stem.

Inability to Eat

The coordination required for swallowing may be damaged after a stroke, or with neurological disorders, or in advanced dementia. There may be damage to the mouth or oesophagus (gullet), from cancer, or from operations to remove cancer. Such damage makes swallowing ineffectual or impossible, and an attempt to swallow will cause distressing gagging or choking.

Problems with Absorption of Nutrients

There may be problems with digestion and absorption of nutrients, associated with a specific illness or because the ageing intestines, like all the other organs of the body, begin to fail. These problems can cause poor nutrition and further loss of appetite in a terminally ill or frail elderly person.

19

Poor Nutrition in Dementia

In Alzheimer's and other types of dementia people reach a stage when they no longer recognise food or know what to do with it. At first they can be spoon fed and their enjoyment or greed indicates that this should be continued. Gradually their taste sensation and feelings of hunger become dulled. They become more withdrawn and do not even respond to the offer of food on a spoon, perhaps taking only one or two mouthfuls and then turning away. In advanced dementia the swallowing reflex is lost and it is impossible to swallow food or water safely. A decision must then be made about artificial hydration and feeding.

Diminishing Appetite

A person who is dying may gradually eat less and less, going from smaller and smaller quantities of solid food to soft food, eventually taking only a few mouthfuls. Even with help, eating becomes more and more exhausting. Some people seem naturally to stop eating almost as a way of finishing their lives when they are close to death.

At a more conscious level, though perhaps making a virtue of necessity, some people regard fasting as a way of controlling death and heightening their spiritual awareness.[4] They eat less, then only soft food, then only fluids, eventually just fruit juices or water. In this way they feel in control as they become weaker and fade away. I am not sure whether this is a conscious decision or a response to the inevitable.

Making the right decision about artificial feeding

I believe there is a fine line between loss of appetite, not being strong enough to eat, and intuitive awareness that death is approaching. In many situations, although the dying person can swallow, they do not take enough fluid or food. A dying person wants less food, and gradually takes less water, even when their swallowing reflex is intact.

Many dying people cannot swallow satisfactorily and are in danger of choking if they are persuaded to take anything by mouth.

So long as they can swallow, a dying person should be offered food and water and helped to eat if they want to. Unfortunately there is evidence that this does not always happen.[5] A study commissioned by *Age Concern* found that some old people in hospital are not given appropriate food, or are not given the time or the help they need to eat. This is one reason why nutrition and artificial feeding in terminal illness is so controversial, and why it is important that a decision is made about which everyone is clear[6].

A healthy person who is denied food or who goes on hunger strike will suffer, even more so if they also do not take fluid. A dying person from whom artificial nutrition is withheld, but who is well nursed, does not suffer from starvation as a healthy person would, because their perception of the need for food is diminished. Nursing care would include giving fluid by a drip – artificial hydration. Simple glucose solution in the drip can maintain the low level of energy input required for a dying person.

PROGRESS OF CHRONIC DISEASE

The next sections describe the end stages of long term disease processes: respiratory disease, heart disease, stroke, cancer and dementia, which lead eventually to the fatal events already described. The path taken from the early stages of a fatal disease to death is called the 'trajectory of disease'[7] (A trajectory is defined as 'the path of an object moving under the action of given forces'). The trajectory of a disease is a major influence on where death takes place: in hospital, in a hospice, a care home or the patient's own home (see Chapter 6).

Respiratory Disease

The lungs can be damaged by smoking, repeated infections, irritation from pollution or industrial processes, or spread of cancer. The lungs lose the elasticity needed to pull air in and push air out of the fine tissues where oxygen and carbon dioxide are exchanged. Not enough oxygen enters the blood stream, and instead carbon dioxide which should be breathed out, accumulates.

Sometimes the air space in the lungs is gradually filled up with fluid. There may be a cancer which exudes fluid, or there may be an infection with lots of sputum, - too much to cough up. Heart failure is a cause of respiratory failure - the heart cannot pump effectively, so fluid backs up in the lungs.

In chronic respiratory disease, the lungs gradually become unable to accept sufficient oxygen into the blood stream. As the lungs absorb less oxygen all the tissues and organs of the body suffer and deteriorate. The patient loses the appetite and energy to eat or even drink enough. They lose weight. At the end, the fingers and feet become blue and consciousness is clouded. Death occurs when the heart or brain stem cease to function due to lack of oxygen.

Heart Disease

With ageing, and especially if there is high blood pressure, the arteries in the muscles of the heart may become narrowed and stiffened. Fatty deposits, atherosclerosis, may build up on the damaged arteries. Education about a healthy lifestyle and effective treatment for diabetes, high blood pressure and raised cholesterol have helped reduce the incidence of heart disease. The vast improvements in treatment of heart disease have reduced the death rate. Therefore the average age of death from heart disease is much older than it used to be.

If the coronary arteries are damaged, the heart muscle may be deprived of oxygen, which causes angina (severe chest pain) and can lead on to a heart attack. A person dying from heart disease may have had one or more heart attacks in the past which have damaged the heart muscle. At any time they may have another heart attack, which may be fatal.

The heart muscle itself can become scarred and stretched thin, in the same way as other muscles of the body also deteriorate visibly with ageing. The thinned heart muscle pumps less efficiently.

Sometimes the valves of the heart start to leak. This can be caused by a heart attack, by a rare viral infection of the heart, or by an inherent weakness of the valve, due to ageing. As other organs deteriorate, toxins that are building up in the blood can interfere with the timing of the heart beat so that it goes too slow or too fast. This timing error can also occur if the area of the heart which initiates each heart beat is damaged.

Damaged muscle, leaking valves or abnormal heart rhythm can cause heart failure as the pumping action becomes less efficient. As the heart fails, congestion builds up in the veins returning the blood to the heart. Fluid collects in the lungs and in the ankles. The failing heart cannot keep up the supply of blood to the lungs to absorb oxygen, or to the other organs to provide oxygen there. All the organs start to deteriorate. The patient becomes ill and exhausted, and may die in their sleep, have a heart attack, or die from respiratory failure as the lungs become more congested.

The Trajectory of Chronic Respiratory Disease and Chronic Heart Disease

The patient is in a poor state of health which continues to decline. Any challenge such as infection anywhere in the body, or over-exertion, can precipitate a life threatening crisis. This crisis could be a heart attack or a sudden severe worsening of heart failure or respiratory failure. This would result in severe breathlessness, wheezing or coughing, which may cause collapse. (Over-exertion in this context means, for example, hurrying to answer the door or having a difficult bowel motion or getting up to fetch a book – not things that would normally be considered over-exertion. People dying from chronic respiratory disease or heart failure may eventually become so breathless they can barely speak and cannot climb the stairs.)

People with any form of severe lung disease or heart disease are susceptible to repeated life threatening chest infections. The whole body is exhausted and the chronic symptoms of cough and breathlessness suddenly become much worse. In each crisis the patient may die, and is more likely to die if they are not admitted to hospital. With hospital treatment they may recover to their former state of gradually declining health. After each episode the heart and lungs are weaker than before and the person may be more disabled by angina and breathlessness.

Frequent episodes occur in which hospital treatment is needed. Each time symptoms are more distressing and the treatment becomes more invasive. In each crisis the likelihood of death increases, but the response to treatment cannot be predicted with certainty. It is difficult to provide the support needed in a community home or the patient's own home - this is why nearly all deaths from chronic heart or respiratory disease occur in hospital.

Stroke

A stroke is caused by loss of the blood supply (ischemia) in part of the brain. The damaged area of the brain is called a stroke or an infarct. (Sometimes slow decline and encroaching dementia is caused by repeated insidious small strokes – this is called 'multi-infarct dementia').

The blood supply may be cut off by a clot forming locally in the sluggish circulation of an artery already damaged by atherosclerosis (see p. 22). Or a damaged artery can split and bleed into part of the brain. Occasionally, a small clot from elsewhere is carried into the brain - a cerebral embolism. The area of the brain supplied by the damaged artery can recover if the circulation quickly gets going again. This transient ischemic attack (TIA) can be the warning sign of a stroke.

If the circulation does not get going again, a significant area of the brain is permanently damaged—a stroke—and the patient is left with a variable degree of disability. A severe stroke often causes paralysis of the arms and/or legs on one side of the body and the opposite side of the face, with difficulties of vision, speech and swallowing.

If the brain stem is damaged by the stroke death can occur suddenly because both breathing and the heartbeat stop. This explains why sometimes a patient may die suddenly at home or soon after admission to hospital.

Paralysis and rigidity of the muscles due to the stroke prevent the patient from moving about so they are prone to deep vein thrombosis leading to pulmonary embolism. They may also develop urinary infection, respiratory infection or pressure ulcers which may lead to blood poisoning. Any of these complications may be fatal.

Time is needed for investigations to give an idea about survival and improvement, and to allow for the possibility of a degree of recovery of mental capacity. Brain scans show the area of damage and are a guide to the likely outcome - the prognosis.

The Trajectory of Stroke
The course of this disease is very variable. Depending on the site and extent of the stroke there may be some recovery, sometimes a good recovery, but with increasing residual damage if further strokes occur.

Hospital admission is required for resuscitation, diagnosis of the extent of the stroke, and nursing care for the sudden severe disabilities, when a stroke occurs. It is increasingly possible to offer thrombolytic drugs 'clotbusters' to dissolve the clots which cause certain strokes, giving a much better outlook. This has to be done within a few hours and is not applicable to all cases of stroke. The FAST campaign (Face Arms Speech Time[8]) aims for early recognition of a stroke and rapid admission to hospital. Treatments are also available routinely which are successful in reducing the risk of further strokes following the initial one.

Many people survive and after rehabilitation are able to return home. They may live for a long time with manageable disabilities, and die eventually from another stroke or from a different disease, not related to the stroke.

A stroke may cause sudden death. Sometimes the patient dies from the complications of stroke, a few hours, days or weeks after admission to hospital, rather than immediately after the stroke.

If the patient survives, other parts of the brain may gradually take over the function of the damaged area and there can be a good recovery. However, as a person ages and becomes less resilient there is less brain capacity for re-learning. Also, the body cannot compensate for weakness in a limb as a younger body would. Mobility, nutrition, self care and motivation are all affected; in this way a stroke contributes to the deterioration of general health.

Some people remain severely disabled after a stroke: unable to speak intelligibly, unable to walk, and unable to manage their personal care, including spectacles and hearing aids.

The cough reflex and the ability to swallow may be disrupted by the stroke. The patient cannot drink so will be given fluids from a drip. Also, they cannot eat and therefore will need artificial nutrition by nasogastric tube. If mental capacity is not regained after some time, the outlook is very poor. By this time the nasogastric tube will be causing irritation and possibly infection. A decision must be made about more invasive artificial nutrition by PEG tube (see p.39). An Advance Decision may take effect - artificial nutrition may be withheld. Artificial hydration through a drip is unlikely to be withheld as it is important for maintaining comfort, though the drip may be withdrawn in the late stages.

Hospital or nursing home are the most frequent place of death from stroke. Hospital because of the urgent initial investigation and treatment, and nursing home because of the high level of care which cannot be provided in their own home, required for people with severe disabilities following stroke.

Cancer

Cancer usually starts in one part of the body, unless it is cancer of the blood forming cells, which is more widespread in the bloodstream from the start. Cancer can spread to other parts of the body, first of all to the local lymph glands (local spread) and then to liver, lung, brain or bones, or other organs. The mode of death will depend on the pattern of growth and spread.

Some problems from cancer are caused by the effects of pressure from the growing tumour. Many structures of the body are tubes – the gut, blood vessels, the urinary system, the airways - and these can all be blocked by pressure from cancer. If the growing cancer presses directly on an organ it can cause abnormal function. Pressure is also the major cause of pain in cancer – pressure on nerves directly or through distortion of other structures.

Growing cancers may produce fluid, some more than others. This fluid is often rich in nutrients, so if a great deal of fluid is produced, this depletes the fluid and nutrients available for normal function of the vital organs. People dying from cancer usually lose weight, and their organs are compromised by poor nutrition. Cancer in the lung secretes fluid which gradually in spite of treatment builds up and causes breathlessness and eventually death from lack of oxygen.

Death from chest infection is common as poor nutrition and the effects of chemotherapy damage the immune system.

Cancer cells replace normal tissues in the body with fragile friable tissues which break down easily. This breakdown is called 'erosion'. The organs and tubal structures of the body have quite strong and supple outer layers, but these can be eroded by the cancer cells so that they leak. For example, erosion into the bowel can cause faeces to leak into the abdominal cavity causing death from overwhelming infection; erosion into a blood vessel causes internal bleeding, which may be fatal.

Spread of cancer to the brain may affect mental capacity and can cause pressure which damages and eventually prevents the vital functions of the brain stem, (see p.16)

The Trajectory of Cancer

Cancer is characterised by long periods of 'living with cancer' intermittently receiving treatment which may have unpleasant side effects. The cancer and its symptoms are brought largely under control. Sometimes an operation is required which may result in some disability, but usually cancer patients are able to go on living at home.

Many cancer patients are completely cured or in remission for many years. If the cancer ceases to respond to treatment, in the end phase of the disease the patient develops more unpleasant symptoms: increased pain, breathlessness and anxiety. It is usually a matter of months during which everyone is aware that death is approaching. Home nursing and hospice services for people dying from cancer are well developed and there is time to plan. Long stays in hospital and death in hospital can usually be avoided.

Dementia

During most of the course of dementia much of the patient's personality may remain intact and there are lots of things in life which they can enjoy. Alzheimer's disease typically lasts several years from diagnosis to death. With earlier diagnosis and better treatment, the early stages, with only mild dementia, will become longer.

In the later stages, death is preceded by a period of withdrawal, immobility and ultimately lack of awareness. Their family suffers grief at the loss of the person they have known, while still wanting to be with them and look after them. As the disease progresses the patient will become unable to feed themselves. Either they no longer recognise food, or they forget how to eat. For a time they may be eager to be spoon-fed, but will eventually cease to be able to swallow as the swallowing reflex is destroyed by the relentless brain damage. The question of artificial feeding will arise.

The patient becomes completely dependent but has no mind with which to direct their care, and in the last stages, no awareness of their environment, or bodily needs, although they still feel pain. The dementia will progress and eventually cause immobility, painful contractions of the muscles and incontinence. It is a triumph of nursing care if pressure ulcers are avoided. Death will finally come from failure of the brain stem or a combination of dehydration, poor nutrition, chest infection and organ failure.

The Trajectory of Dementia

The course of dementia is to some extent predictable, although many people with dementia die from another disease, since dying from dementia takes several years from diagnosis.

At first there is anxiety, poor organisation of tasks, forgetfulness and loss of concentration. For several years the quality of life is reasonable. The person with dementia is aware that they are

29

gradually losing their mind, but they are able to enjoy life between episodes of fear, grief, confusion and panic. These feelings of enjoyment and despair are mirrored in the carer, usually the husband or wife.

Most carers are heroic, but people with dementia usually reach a stage when they can no longer be cared for at home. Depending on the circumstances, this may be months or even years before death. The reasons care at home breaks down are illness or exhaustion of the main carer, verbal or physical abuse directed at the carer, or inability of the carer to maintain an acceptable level of care due to the constant complex needs of the person with dementia. Most difficult is the maintenance of hygiene and dignity in the presence of faecal incontinence.

Most people who die from dementia die in a care home or nursing home. The trajectory is one of slow relentless decline to a state of complete dependency which may persist for months before death. Many end their days being artificially fed.

Dying from Old Age

Some people die from the gradual deterioration of ageing. They have many health problems, but no one disease predominates. They become increasingly frail, sometimes retaining mental acuity, more often becoming somewhat confused and forgetful. They have a series of hospital admissions, perhaps for a chest or urinary infection, or a minor stroke or heart attack, but after treatment, continue as before in gradual decline.

Such frail old people are often single by now, having survived their husband or wife. They require more and more care, and often end their lives in a care home. There they are usually well looked after, kept warm and nourished, while they gradually fade away. At the end, a doctor will identify for the death certificate one of their many problems as the cause of death – usually heart failure or respiratory failure.

This death is not the same as one from severe established chronic heart or respiratory disease. A doctor might want to put 'old age' on the death certificate as cause of death, but although acceptable this is discouraged. It is preferred that the doctor makes a specific diagnosis as this contributes to statistics which are used for developing and monitoring the impact of public health education and medical interventions.

PALLIATIVE CARE[9]

'Palliative Care is the active holistic care of patients with advanced progressive illness. Management of pain and other symptoms and provision of psychological, social and spiritual support is paramount. The goal of palliative care is achievement of the best quality of life for patients and their families. Palliative care is ideally introduced when it becomes clear that the patient and their family face a life threatening illness.'[9]

Palliative care aims to:

Affirm life and regard dying as a normal process;

Provide relief from pain and other distressing symptoms;

Integrate the psychological and spiritual aspects of care;

Support patients to live as actively as possible until death;

Support the family during the patient's illness and in bereavement.

The needs of the patient and their family are recorded and updated by all the different people providing care. They record and share information in this way so that everyone understands what the problems are and how the patient's day to day palliative care is aimed at ameliorating each problem so that death is as dignified and peaceful as possible (see pp. 7).

What are the Last Days Like?

The last days of life often follow a similar pattern. Drugs may be stopped now which the patient has been taking for many years:- such as Aspirin, cholesterol lowering drugs, medication for blood pressure, etc. The patient's comfort is the main concern, so medicines which help to maintain comfort or prevent symptoms will not be withdrawn.

Doctors and nurses will consider whether any further investigations or tests (even simple actions such as taking the patient's temperature or blood pressure) would be helpful, or just intrusive.

The patient is usually bed bound by this time, or propped up in a chair during the day. Their position will be adjusted often, to maintain comfort and prevent pressure sores.

They may take sips of water and possibly welcome small amounts of food, or eat nothing. Mouth care will be provided. (Some illnesses cause under or overproduction of saliva.) A patient who cannot swallow will be given fluids and perhaps glucose solution through a drip. At the very last a drip may be removed, or replaced by a shunt which enables drugs to be given gradually by a continuous syringe pump, often into a vein in the neck.

They can receive oxygen through a face mask or nasal tubes, to help them to remain conscious and reduce breathlessness so that they can talk.

The dying person will pass very little urine or faeces. Soiling is managed by using absorbent pads. They will be bathed every day. Retention of urine, or constipation, may cause agitation, but usually these problems can be helped by catheterisation or the judicious use of drugs.

The dying person will become weaker, sleep more and breathe

less deeply. Sometimes they will stop breathing for short periods, or take several rapid deep breaths. Their cough becomes ineffectual and secretions in the windpipe may 'rattle' – the 'death rattle'. Fingers and toes become blue as the circulation fails.

A dying person may need strong medication to relieve their symptoms. Morphine is often used to control pain, breathlessness and anxiety. Drugs may be needed to prevent possible side effects of morphine - vomiting and constipation. Another side effect is hallucinations. If side effects are troublesome, alternatives to morphine can be used.

If symptoms become more difficult to control, the dying person may be anxious and agitated. Sedation may be introduced. Initially the aim is to allow periods of lucidity, but if the suffering is too much the sedation can be deepened. In a few people this deep sedation is the only way of relieving severe symptoms.

In 2007 international palliative care experts agreed that 'terminal sedation would be appropriate when death is very close and other treatments fail to relieve symptoms'.[11] Carefully judged doses of sedative and morphine are given to ensure that the dying person is comfortable as their life comes to a close.

In the majority of people, the impact of symptoms becomes less as their consciousness becomes clouded, and they drift away peacefully into death.

REFERENCES

1. Henry King (1592-1669). *A Contemplation Upon Flowers.* The Metaphysical Poets. Ed: Helen Gardner. London, Penguin 1957.

2. Deaths registered in England and Wales (Series DR). Death rates per million population. *Table 5*. Office for National Statistics 2015.

3. *End of Life Care.* National Audit Office. Stationery Office, 2008.

4. Nearing H. *At the End of a Good Life: Scott Nearing's dignified death sets an inspiring example for us all.* In Context; 26: Summer 1990.

5. *Hungry to be Heard: The scandal of malnourished people in hospital.* Age Concern 2006.

6. Hassain M, Durrani S. *Looking for Guidance: dementia and PEG tube feeding.* Geriatric Medicine; October 2005.

7. Murray SA, Kendall M, Boyd K, Sheik A. *Illness Trajectories and Palliative Care.* British Medical Journal 2005; 330: 1007-1011.

8. *What is the FAST test?* Web site: stroke.org.uk/ I need information. Stroke Association UK. 2015.

9. *Definition of Palliative Care* The National Council for Palliative care 2012

10. Murray A, Boyd K, Byock I. *Continuous deep sedation in patients nearing death.* British Medical Journal 2008; 336: 781-782.

Chapter 3

Life Sustaining Treatments

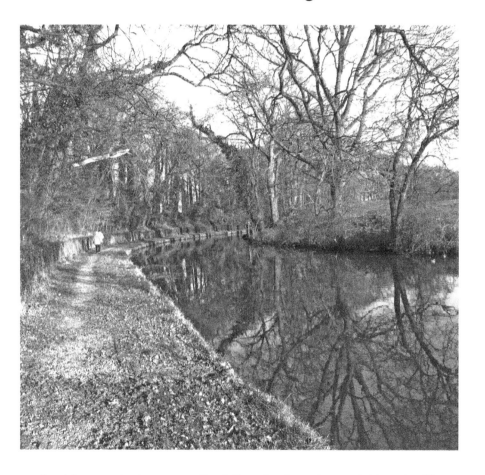

And is one to be sorry that the doctors brought her to life
and operated, or not?

Simone de Beauvoir (1908-1986)

A person is kept alive by supporting, taking over, or bypassing the functions of the body - in other words - by 'life-sustaining treatments'. An Advance Decision to Refuse Treatment comes into effect if you have lost the mental capacity to take part in discussions about your treatment. In it you describe those circumstances in which you refuse life-sustaining treatment even though this may hasten your death.

Although an Advance Decision is legally binding it is not a complete 'hands off' to doctors. They must decide about your mental capacity and whether the clinical circumstances are applicable. Two situations are worth noting:

Life -sustaining treatments in an emergency

In an emergency - in sudden illness such as a heart attack, or after an accident, immediate active treatment is the rule. If you are unconscious and dying, doctors and nurses will attempt to resuscitate you. They will not stop to read your Advance Decision. 'Treatment must be provided which is the least restrictive of the patient's future options'[2].

Life-sustaining treatment may be withheld or withdrawn later, in accordance with an Advance Decision, after investigations to assess mental capacity, confirm the diagnosis of terminal illness and evaluate proposed treatment options. A Do Not Attempt to Resuscitate agreement (see pp. 83, 89, 100) is more appropriate if you wish to refuse emergency cardiopulmonary resuscitation.

Life -sustaining Treatment and Palliative Care

A treatment which may prolong life can sometimes be the best way to keep a person comfortable: continuing with established medication to alleviate breathlessness in heart or respiratory disease; antibiotics for a painful infection; maintaining hydration with an intravenous drip; chemotherapy or radiotherapy to reduce painful pressure by reducing the size of a cancer; and other treatments, always depending on the needs of a particular patient.

The aim is for my death to be free of severe pain and anxiety, and not prolonged. Therefore I have refused 'treatments aimed *purely* at sustaining my life' in my Advance Decision, not excluding treatments which may slightly prolong my life, but which may be used because such treatment happens to be the best way of controlling pain or unpleasant symptoms.

LIFE SUSTAINING TREATMENTS

ARTIFICIAL HYDRATION – THE INTRAVENOUS DRIP

Artificial hydration is usually given by a drip. Fluid from a bag is allowed to drip steadily into a vein in the arm, through a thin flexible tube, called a cannula.

When someone cannot swallow, they cannot eat or drink. Conditions in which the ability to swallow is lost are described in the previous chapter. The need for water or other fluid is immediate. The patient may die very quickly from shock or within a few days from dehydration. The decision about artificial hydration must be made immediately or within hours, (whereas the decision about artificial nutrition can wait for a few days.)

In a conscious patient the ability to swallow is assessed by the speech and language therapist (SALT). They are the right people to do this because many of the nerves and muscles used in speech are also used in chewing and swallowing. When someone is unconscious this assessment is not appropriate. A drip will be started, and their ability to swallow liquids can be tested when consciousness returns.

Is a Drip Part of Ordinary Nursing Care?

A drip is not usually invasive or burdensome. It is important to doctors and nurses because as well as maintaining hydration (although to a limited extent), it helps them to treat unpleasant symptoms by giving drugs directly into a vein, when the patient cannot swallow. Also, a low level of energy can be provided by giving a simple glucose solution via a drip.

As a person dies the sensation of thirst diminishes. Their mouth can be moistened and if they can swallow a little, sips of water are given. They do not die of 'thirst' as you might imagine it. At death most people have become dehydrated. This is not because sufficient fluid has been deliberately or carelessly withheld. It is because, close to death, the kidneys and the heart would be overloaded by normal amounts of fluid.

A drip is part of ordinary nursing care required to keep a person comfortable. Though it may prolong life it is not aimed 'purely at prolonging life', therefore it is not precluded by my Advance Decision.

Problems with a Drip

The veins in a frail old person are fragile and with a drip may tend to split or to clot. When this happens, the fluid seeps into the surrounding flesh of the arm and can cause bruising and swelling, sometimes damaging the skin.

It is not uncommon for a person who is dying to pull out their drip in confusion and agitation. Usually the drip can be moved to another site perhaps less noticeable to the patient.

If necessary, another means of giving fluid can be established – into the soft flexible skin of the abdomen. The fluid spreads and is absorbed through the tissues underneath the skin, but it is not possible to give as much fluid this way and the amount of fluid absorbed is unpredictable.

An alternative to a drip is a syringe pump (used to give continuous pain relief and sedation at the end of life) with a fine cannula inserted into a vein in the neck.

ARTIFICIAL NUTRITION

This is perhaps the most controversial element of the care of dying people, especially those who have lost mental capacity.[3] Someone who cannot swallow can receive nutrients through a drip for a time, or nutrition can be provided by a tube – either through the nose and throat into the stomach (a nasogastric tube) or, if that is not tolerated or if it is repeatedly pulled out by the patient, the tube must go directly into the stomach. A flange is placed on the front of the abdomen, through which a tube goes through the abdomen into the stomach (a percutaneous endogastric (PEG) tube). This PEG tube is guided into place aided by an endoscopy, using a fibre-optic tube into the stomach via the mouth.

Artificial feeding may be considered in a number of circumstances in a terminally ill person. The NHS has been criticised for allowing elderly patients to become malnourished while in hospital,[4] therefore doctors and nurses will want to avoid this criticism being levelled at them. If the patient cannot swallow or if adequate nutrition cannot be provided by spoon-feeding because the patient becomes exhausted, doctors and nurses will be inclined to start artificial feeding.

An Advance Decision will help in discussions about providing or withholding artificial nutrition. If artificial nutrition is to be withheld the family will need to be reassured that allowing the patient to die in this way will not involve terrific hunger and suffering. Appetite often gradually diminishes to nothing when a person is dying. A drip may be continued to provide hydration and small amounts of nutrients until death is imminent.

WHEN MIGHT A PERSON BE ARTIFICIALLY FED?

Artificial Nutrition Post Operatively

Surgical operations are discussed on p.48.
If the patient is unable to eat following an operation, they may

require artificial feeding for a time. This should be explained beforehand as the patient should give informed consent to the operation. After the operation it may take a while for the patient to regain consciousness and they may lack mental capacity initially, but there is usually a few days grace before the decision about artificial nutrition has to be made.

If mental capacity is not regained, and the patient still cannot eat, after a certain point, if artificial feeding is further delayed, there will be rapid deterioration. Doctors may decide that having undergone the operation the patient would expect everything including artificial feeding to be done to help them to recover. If not, why operate? This is a matter of judgement. Sincerely wanting to do the best for the patient, sometimes a doctor may err on the side of mistaken optimism. (See p. 51.)

Artificial Nutrition In Cancer of the Mouth, Throat or Oesophagus

Cancer in this area may prevent the patient from swallowing normally. An operation may allow the person to swallow, but initially the operation itself, or other treatment, results in inability to swallow. This inability may be temporary, with recovery expected and aided by artificial nutrition.

Most cancer patients will be mentally capable and able to decide for themselves whether such an operation, with its inevitable postoperative difficulties, requiring artificial nutrition and possibly ventilation, would be acceptable. Communication might be difficult, the patient might not be able to speak because of the site of the cancer, but they must be enabled to communicate their wishes in other ways.

For a patient who is not mentally capable, an Advance Decision would indicate whether in these circumstances they would wish to refuse an operation.

Artificial Nutrition After Head Injury

If unconsciousness persists, after about two weeks of feeding by nasogastric tube, doctors and relatives must decide whether to establish ongoing artificial feeding by PEG tube.

A terminally ill or frail elderly person has a poor prognosis after severe head injury. Doctors may decide to allow the patient to die on the grounds that continuing treatment would be invasive and burdensome, out of proportion to any possible benefit, with little likelihood of restoring mental capacity. This is a difficult decision for doctors to make especially if that person was previously mentally capable. An Advance Decision to Refuse Treatment enables the family to engage in discussion about the aims and possible outcome of treatment, at an early stage, helped by a clear expression of what the patient's wishes would be.

A previously well person who has recently lost mental capacity as a result of brain injury presents a particular problem if loss of consciousness is persistent. This is especially so as these injuries, though rare, are more common among young people. Less invasive life sustaining treatments such as artificial nutrition by nasogastric tube, and ventilation by endotracheal tube would be started, but after about two weeks, if unconsciousness persists, more invasive, ongoing life sustaining treatment such as PEG feeding and/or ventilation by endotracheal tube (see p. 47) would be needed.

Once established these can only be withdrawn after application to the High Court.[5] The dilemma presented by prolonged unconsciousness and need for invasive life support in a previously well person is discussed on p. 71. In my own Advance Decision I have used wording which stops short of an outright refusal of invasive treatment, but asks for life support to be withheld if any possible benefit (taking into account my age) is outweighed by a high risk of living on with severe mental and physical disability.

Artificial Nutrition After a Stroke

A stroke can damage the part of the brain stem which controls the swallowing reflex so the patient cannot eat. Artificial nutrition may be introduced because the prognosis of a stroke is often unclear initially. Improvement can be dramatic especially if plenty of healthy brain tissue remains. This will show on the brain scan. Improvement is less likely if large areas of the brain are already damaged due to earlier strokes, or if the new stroke is massive.

If there is severe damage, perhaps on top of previous strokes, and the patient is already elderly and frail, it is unlikely mental capacity will be recovered. The patient's Advance Decision will indicate refusal of artificial nutrition.

Dementia and Artificial Nutrition

People with dementia may not recognise food in front of them and forget how to feed themselves. If they have an appetite they must be spoon fed. Later they may start refusing to open their mouth, turn away, or refuse to swallow. Even though their swallowing reflex might still be intact, they accept less and less food.

The patient becomes more likely to choke on food, and eventually unable to swallow due to inexorable brain damage affecting the brain stem. Research evidence suggests that artificial nutrition in dementia does not improve either quality of life or survival.[6]

Pacemakers

Though a pacemaker will reduce your risk of dying it is not solely or even mainly a life-sustaining treatment. Its main effect is to make you more comfortable. Most pacemakers are the size of a matchbox, inserted under local anaesthetic beneath the skin of the chest with little post operative discomfort. They provide electrical impulses to the heart to keep the heartbeat regular. The improvement in the circulation ensures better delivery of oxygen to the organs and tissues of the body, so the unpleasant symptoms caused by an irregular heartbeat are improved. A person who lacks mental capacity is still capable of feeling physically better, and improved circulation may improve mental functioning for a time, so a pacemaker, if clinically indicated, will probably be a good idea.

Antibiotics

The choice of whether or not to give antibiotics could depend on the characteristics of the infection as well as factors to do with the patient. If clinical isolation and barrier nursing are not available, certain infections must be treated with antibiotics as a matter of public health to stop spread of infection to other people. These considerations might override an Advance Decision.

Localised infections are painful, and not likely to be fatal. A patient with dementia, who had an infected finger or a mild lower urinary tract infection would be treated with antibiotics in order to make them more comfortable - a means to prevent suffering rather than a life sustaining treatment.

In a severe chest infection, antibiotics would be regarded as life sustaining treatment, to be withheld in accordance with an Advance Decision, if the patient had permanently lost mental capacity and was terminally ill.

Blood Transfusion

For some religious groups blood transfusion is unacceptable. This is respected when a mentally capable adult refuses transfusion. A person who refuses blood transfusion on religious grounds can write an Advance Decision with specific detailed instructions refusing blood transfusion under any circumstances.

There are many circumstances in which doctors would hope that mental capacity could be restored by active treatment including blood transfusion: after blood loss due to trauma or operation;

in leukemia; in chronic anemia due to poor diet or hidden blood loss. If someone who lacks mental capacity is given a necessary blood transfusion for any of the above reasons, just like anyone else they will feel better and less breathless, and mental function may improve.

If there is doubt about whether blood transfusion is in the patient's best interest, the doctor will discuss it with colleagues and the patient's family, guided by an Advance Decision if there is one. In circumstances of severe haemorrhage due to cancer erosion, blood transfusion would be invasive. Morphine would be given to ease the patient's inevitable death.

Renal Dialysis

Dialysis is a means of purifying the patient's bloodstream of substances normally excreted by the kidneys. It is a life-sustaining treatment for renal failure. Dialysis is performed by a renal dialysis machine (artificial kidney) or by peritoneal dialysis.

For renal dialysis by machine a plastic tube is used to make a loop between an artery and a vein in the patient's arm so that blood can be taken from their body into the dialysis machine and back into their body. In the machine, the blood is passed over a membrane which absorbs the toxic substances which the kidney would normally remove. The blood returning to the body is then free of these toxins.

For peritoneal dialysis the patient's abdominal cavity is filled with a quantity of sterile fluid. This fluid absorbs the toxins across the lining of the abdominal cavity which is called the peritoneum - hence 'peritoneal dialysis'. It can be used as a short term measure until a dialysis machine becomes available, or to allow time for damaged kidneys to recover, for example after an infection. A person who is unconscious can receive dialysis to prevent clinical deterioration.

Dialysis would be appropriate for an elderly person with mental capacity, if other organs were functioning normally. Dialysis would be inappropriate and therefore probably not suggested for a person who had permanently lost mental capacity and would be unable to understand or tolerate the procedure. An Advance Decision would help the family to accept that the patient would not have wished for dialysis in these circumstances.

TREATMENTS FOR RESPIRATORY FAILURE
Oxygen

The initial treatment for respiratory failure is with an oxygen mask or nasal tubes which provide a constant stream of oxygen and air at ordinary atmospheric pressure. It is not unduly invasive or burdensome and will make a person with respiratory failure more comfortable. It could be regarded as an example of ordinary nursing care. It is not primarily life sustaining. It will not help with expulsion of carbon dioxide, and can be exhausting as the respiratory muscles must do all the work. Someone dying from respiratory disease needs more than an oxygen mask for their life to be prolonged significantly.

Noninvasive Ventilation (Respiratory Support)

In spite of respiratory relieving drugs, and oxygen and air, and antibiotics (if appropriate), the patient may still not obtain enough oxygen. Noninvasive mechanical ventilation will be proposed. This is widely used for patients with respiratory failure due to lung disease or heart failure, and has recently been recommended by NICE [7] to support the breathing of patients with Motor Neurone Disease.

Bi-level Positive Airways Pressure

A mask over the nose and mouth is connected to an air pump. The airflow is strongest as you breathe in, so you take in as much air as possible. There is less pressure when you breathe out, but

45

enough to keep the airways open. The machine helps with the muscular effort of breathing and with the expulsion of carbon dioxide as well as intake of air.

This treatment is suitable for patients who are conscious and able to tolerate and cooperate with it, and who have a sufficiently strong cough to expel phlegm when needed. A person who can calm themselves and is strong enough to cooperate may do well; in a later crisis when they are more frail the same person may experience claustrophobia and fear, and fight against the machine. Sedation may be needed, but this can increase disorientation or cause drowsiness or unconsciousness. At this point doctors may decide on ventilation.

After several experiences of positive airways pressure a person who is increasingly disabled with respiratory failure may decide that next time they would rather be allowed to die. Detailed instructions in the Advance Decision could refuse positive pressure ventilation. Suitable wording is given on the Motor Neurone Disease website[8]. However the MND Society suggest it would be a mistake to tie doctors hands with regard to treatment unless you are very sure, in which case a Do Not Attempt to Resuscitate agreement might be more appropriate.

Ventilation by endotracheal tube
Ventilation by endotracheal tube is routine during operations requiring a general anaesthetic. A tube is passed through the mouth into the throat and windpipe, and removed later as the patient regains consciousness.

Ventilation of an unconscious patient, by endotracheal tube, is required in many emergency situations: accident, a head injury or stroke, or a heart attack. The endotracheal tube can usually be maintained until the patient regains consciousness and can breathe spontaneously again.

Ventilation via tracheostomy?

In a conscious patient an endotracheal tube could not be tolerated in the throat because of the gag reflex. In a patient who remains unconscious an endotracheal tube can be maintained for a limited period, about two weeks, before it begins to cause damage to the lining of the throat and becomes a focus for infection.

Therefore if continued ventilation is required to sustain life, a tracheostomy is created. Under general anaesthesia a plastic tube is inserted directly through the front of the neck into the lower part of the throat, bypassing the mouth and throat and delivering oxygen straight to the windpipe and into the lungs. This is less irritant than an endotracheal tube and can be maintained into the future.

No air passes across the voice box which is in the throat above the tracheostomy. If the muscles of the voice box are still working it is possible to speak but with difficulty - the tracheostomy tube must be temporarily closed off with a finger or pad.

In some situations, for example after stroke or severe brain injury, it takes time to establish the probable outcome of treatment, so a tracheostomy may be needed if the patient cannot breathe spontaneously. In due course, if the patient has terminal disease and is not likely to recover mental capacity an Advance Decision would come into effect and the ventilator would be switched off.

Ventilation may therefore allow the relatives some time to say goodbye to the patient. This can be valuable even though the patient remains unconscious.

Life sustaining treatment and severe head injury

Severe head injuries and catastrophic strokes can result in persistent unconsciousness. Even if the person was previously healthy, the outlook is poor if unconsciousness persists for some time.

Nasogastric tube feeding and an endotracheal tube for ventilation become unsustainable after about two weeks due to irritation and infection, so if the patient is to live, invasive ongoing life support measures are needed:- PEG tube feeding and/or a tracheostomy for assisted ventilation.

The hope in starting invasive treatment in persistent unconsciousness is that the patient will improve. They may eventually regain consciousness and mental capacity. They may have disabilities but with support can live a meaningful life. In general, the longer a person is unconscious the worse the prognosis, but this is by no means universal.

Brain injury may be so severe that although the body can be kept alive, there is minimal brain activity. The patient is not 'brain dead' but they are in a persistent vegetative state (PSV) where there is no awareness of the self or the environment, no purposeful behaviours and no comprehension or significant expression.

Therefore where brain injury is very severe and as time passes there is no improvement, a decision must be made whether or not to embark upon invasive life support. This watershed, after about two weeks, between non-invasive life support, and moving to invasive measures, is the subject of an article 'the window of opportunity for death after severe brain injury'.[9] It is an opportunity for frank and realistic discussion with the patient's family.

In the article[9] just referred to, the authors described interviews with patients' families, who on returning to the hospital after a short absence had discovered invasive life support measures in place which they had not been consulted about. The situation had shifted from thinking it might be best to allow the patient to die, by withdrawing treatment, to supporting ongoing bodily life, which the patient might not have chosen.

If PSV is diagnosed doctors and families face difficult emotional and ethical problems later in withdrawing established life support. This question is particularly poignant if the person is young.[5] The parents or family must apply to the High Court for a direction to switch off the ventilator and/or withdraw other life support such as PEG feeding.[11]

It has been suggested that an Advance Decision might include a specific direction to refuse life sustaining treatment if after severe head injury unconsciousness persists for two weeks[10] without improvement. However, guidance from the Royal College of Physicians[11] suggests that diagnosis of persistent vegetative state requires more time for observation of signs of recovery, and a number of complex investigations of brain activity. Two weeks may be too soon a cut off point.

In my Advance Decision I have not mentioned a precise duration of persistent unconsciousness but asked my family to balance the possibility of meaningful recovery against the disaster (to me) of ongoing life with severe mental and probably physical disabilities. My Advance Decision and my Statement of Values will enable doctors to make the decision to withhold or withdraw invasive life sustaining treatment. (See pp. 39, 72). What you say about this in your Advance Decision is very personal.[12]

Life-sustaining Operations

In 1999 the topic of the National Confidential Enquiry into Post Operative Deaths (NCEPOD) was 'Extremes of Age'[13], looking at post-operative deaths in people aged 90 years and over. Almost half the deaths occurred on the same or the next day after operation, the remainder within thirty days. These operations caused more suffering than if the patients had been allowed to die with their pain and other symptoms controlled by palliative care.

Perhaps, especially in the very elderly, there is a temptation to be over optimistic about the outcome. This would not matter so much if it were not for the terrible state in which some patients live out their last days post-operatively - on ventilators and monitors, artificially fed and with their wounds unhealed.

In 2005, NCEPOD chose to look at a group of patients for whom the decision *against* surgery had been made.[14.] These were frail elderly patients with an emergency life threatening condition, ruptured aortic aneurysm, where the main blood vessel from the heart has split, causing severe internal bleeding. A total of 78 patients, average age 83 years, were not operated on but given palliative care instead. All of these died peacefully without having to suffer the pain and indignity of an operation.

There were 68 people aged over 80 years who had the same condition, and were operated on. Thirty seven of these were dead within 30 days. The whole panoply of gruelling life sustaining treatments would have been used in the attempt to keep them alive. Only 31 survived more than 30 days. NCEPOD has no data on their quality of life or how long they survived. Was operation the right decision for them?

Operations can benefit old people
Many elective operations benefit elderly people. In people aged over 75 years hip replacements, operations for cancer, coronary bypass surgery, cardiac valve repair and repairs of aortic aneurysm have a successful outcome.

Points to discuss if an operation is proposed
NCEPOD commented: 'Decisions about major surgery on elderly patients are very difficult. Biological not chronological age is the key to good decision making. Biological age is assessed by lung function and cardiac fitness tests, the presence of risk factors

such as obesity, high blood pressure or diabetes, and lifestyle: diet, smoking and exercise.

A patient with mental capacity can chose for themselves and consent to, or refuse the operation. If the patient lacks mental capacity, the surgeon and anaesthetist must consider to what extent mental capacity and a reasonable quality of life might be restored by the operation. If the operation goes ahead, they must make sure that appropriate post operative care will be available.

If the patient cannot be resuscitated before the operation, the outcome is likely to be poor. Emergency operations 'to save the patients life' may, in the nature of things, be futile. If they are going to die anyway, patients might prefer not to have the operation. NCEPOD has recommended against futile surgery in the past'.

An elderly person who is already sick has little resilience to complications such as blood loss, infection, shock, oxygen depletion and dehydration. People with established dementia are at risk of deterioration in mental and physical function as a result of an operation. If it goes ahead, the patient may well live, but remain confused and brain damaged as a result of the lack of an adequate blood supply to the brain, before or during the operation. NCEPOD recommended a specialist in palliative care should be involved so that alternatives to surgery can be considered.

REFERENCES

1. Simone de Beauvoir (1908-1986). *A Very Easy Death.* London, Penguin 1965.

2. The Lord Chancellor. *The Mental Capacity Act Code of Practice.* Department of Constitutional Affairs 2007.

3. Hassain M, Durrani S. *Looking for Guidance: dementia and PEG tube feeding.* Geriatric Medicine, October 2005.

4. *Hungry to Be Heard: The scandal of malnourished people in hospital.* Age Concern 2006.

5. Airedale NHS Trust v. Bland (1993) I All ER821; Law Hospital NHS Trust V. Lord Advocate 1996 SLT 848.

6. Sanders DS, Anderson AJ, Bardhan KD. *Percutaneous endoscopic gastrostomy: an effective strategy for gastrostomy feeding in patients with dementia.* Clinical Medicine 2004; 4: 235-41.

7. *The use of non invasive ventilation in the management of Motor Neurone Disease.* Guidance/cg105. National Institute of Clinical Excellence. Website nice.org.uk 2015.

8. *Advance Decisions to Refuse Treatment.* Information sheet No. 19 Motor Neurone Disease Association. Website MND.org.uk 2015.

9. Kitzinger J, Kitzinger C. *The 'window of opportunity' for death after severe brain injury: family experiences.* Sociology of Health and Illness ISSN 0141-9889,pp1-18; 2012.

10. *Guidance notes and form for an Advance Decision.* Compassion in Dying 2014. Website compassionindying. org.uk.

11. *The Vegetative States: guidance on diagnosis and management.* Royal College of Physicians 2003

Life Sustaining Treatments

12. Rull, G *Vegetative States*. Patient.co.uk 2013.

13. Callum KG, Gray AJG, Hoile RW, Ingram GS, Martin IC, Sherry KM, Whimster F. *Extremes of Age*. National Confidential Enquiry into Peri-Operative Deaths 1999.

14. Hargreaves C, Gray A, Lansdown M, Horrocks M, Rose J, Cunningham A, Black A. *Abdominal aortic aneurysm: a service in need of surgery?* National Confidential Enquiry into Patient Outcomes and Death 2005.

Chapter 4
Living Wills and the
Advance Decision to Refuse Treatment

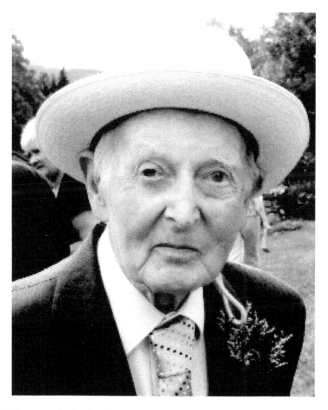

With equal mind, what happens, let us bear,
Nor joy nor grieve too much for things beyond our care,
Like pilgrims to th'appointed place we tend;
The world's an inn, and death the journey's end.

John Dryden (1631-1700)

A n Advance Decision is a document or letter you write when
you are of sound mind, giving guidance and directions about
your medical care, should you in future lose the mental capacity
to take part in discussions with the doctors and nurses looking
after you. In this chapter the Advance Decision is introduced. I
describe the meaning of mental capacity and the lack of it, under
the Mental Capacity Act 2005[2]. Then comes 'How to Write Your
Advance Decision', followed by my own Advance Decision. The
last section is about Lasting Power of Attorney and the Court of
Protection.

The term *living will* covers three different options.[3] These are: a
Statement of Values; an *Advance Directive*; and an *Advance Decision
to Refuse Treatment*.

Statement of Values
This is a written or verbal statement which describes the *motivation
and background for my Advance Decision*. This should be an integral
part of your Advance Decision. You will find my own Statement
of Values, as an example, at the end of my Advance Decision. (My
statement of values also includes my preferences for my personal
care, wishes for my body after death and funeral ceremony.)

The Advance Directive
This was replaced by the Advance Decision under the Mental
Capacity Act. Any Advance Directive still has legal standing and
must be taken into account in treatment decisions.[4]

The Advance Decision to Refuse Treatment
An Advance Decision to Refuse Treatment is a document written
when you have mental capacity. In future if you have lost mental
capacity, it can be used to refuse consent to medical treatment and
thereby avoid having your life prolonged in circumstances when
you would prefer to be allowed to die. It directs that in clinical
circumstances which you describe, treatment which is purely

aimed at sustaining your life should be withheld or withdrawn, even though your life is at risk.

What if there is no Advance Decision?

Doctors caring for you are bound to follow the GMC Guidance on treatment and care towards the end of life:[5]

To start any necessary treatment which is considered to be of some benefit, while the patient's mental capacity is being determined.

To consider whether the patient is in the end stage of a disease or condition and whether death is expected within hours or days or over a longer duration.

To evaluate possibilities for treatment and the likely benefits, burdens and risks of treatment.

To obtain a second opinion from a senior clinician.

To consult those close to the patient for information and to ascertain whether the patient has previously expressed their wishes in an Advance Decision.

So, at the end of life, doctors have a duty to refrain from treatment which is unduly invasive or burdensome to the extent that the patient's suffering outweighs any possible benefit.[5]

With or without an Advance Decision, a senior doctor may decide that an attempt at resuscitation or other life prolonging treatment should be withheld or withdrawn if it is likely to prove futile or if the patient is in the final stages of terminal disease[6.]

The difference with an Advance Decision

An Advance Decision can enable discussions between doctors and nurses and a patients family, which might otherwise be difficult to get started. Who wants to be the first to suggest that treatment

57

be withheld? With an Advance Decision, these discussions cannot be avoided.

My Advance Decision allows me to state the circumstances in which I would prefer treatment to focus on peace and comfort rather than trying to sustain and prolong my life. It will empower my family to question what the aims of my treatment should be.

Doctors recognise the legal right of an adult to refuse consent to treatment. If you lose mental capacity it is only by an Advance Decision that you can express this legal right.

Your Advance Decision provides the opportunity to think about situations that you would find intolerable, and to discuss your feelings and wishes with your family. Then, if you should develop dementia or lose mental capacity, due to accident, or other illness your family will know what your wishes would be.

Your Advance Decision has legal standing and must be taken into account and discussed with colleagues and your family. When a patient lacks mental capacity, doctors and nurses must consider what they and the rest of the health care team know about the patient's wishes, feelings, beliefs and values.[4]

'Failure to give due weight to an Advance Decision can result in loss of a doctor's licence to practise medicine'[5]: the loss of their livelihood and reputation.

A doctor who acts contrary to a valid and applicable Advance Decision may be sued for criminal negligence or assault[7] if a specific treatment that had been refused was administered in specific circumstances which the patient had described. With detailed instructions the Advance Decision can be 'legally binding'. There are pros and cons to detailed instructions, which are discussed in detail (see p. 87-91). They are not particularly helpful at the bedside.

You can write an Advance Decision initially, while you are well, without detailed instructions. An example is my own Advance Decision (see p.73). Later, if you have been diagnosed with a particular disease, you can add optional detailed instructions as the disease progresses, but only if you retain mental capacity. Examples of progressive diseases where mental capacity is retained are cancer, heart failure and respiratory failure, motor neurone disease, Parkinson's disease, HIV, diabetes.

Could I be allowed to die when I had not intended it?

There are safeguards to ensure doctors do not hastily decide to withhold treatment, or allow a patient to deteriorate or die in circumstances the patient did not anticipate when they made their Advance Decision. 'Treatment must be provided to prevent the patient's clinical condition from deteriorating while an apparent Advance Decision is assessed.'[7]

An Advance Decision will not usually prevent emergency resuscitation. Unless there is already a Do Not Attempt to Resuscitate (DNAR) agreement (Ch.5), treatment must be provided to keep the patient's options open, as far as possible.[7]

Time is needed for assessment of mental capacity, and for evaluation of the clinical circumstances - the diagnosis and expected response to treatment. This can be helped if the family or GP are there to inform about your mental capacity and medical history prior to this emergency event, but in an emergency treatment may be started before these people even know you are in hospital. Life sustaining treatment can be withdrawn or withheld later in accordance with an Advance Decision (see p. 36).

An Advance Decision can lead on to a DNAR agreement if doctors agree that it is now appropriate to refrain from any attempt at resuscitation, should cardiac or respiratory arrest or other immediately life threatening event occur.

THE MENTAL CAPACITY ACT

Legal Definition of a Lack of Mental Capacity

Mental capacity is legally defined and is assessed according to guidelines issued by the General Medical Council (GMC) and by the British Medical Association and the Law Society.[8] The legal definition[2] is:

'a person lacks mental capacity if they are unable by reason of mental disability to make a decision on the matter in question or unable to communicate a decision because unconscious or for any other reason. Mental disability is any disability or disorder of the mind or brain, whether permanent or temporary, which results in an impairment or disturbance of mental functioning'.

This legal definition gives rise to the Two Part Test

Assessment of Mental Capacity - The Two Part Test

Part 1: Is there a Disorder or Disability of the Mind or Brain?

Some people never attain sufficient mental capacity to make complex decisions, for example, people with severe learning disabilities from childhood. With most people, capacity is attained as they grow up to adulthood, but may be subsequently lost.

Incapacity may be temporary, due to alcohol or drugs; or capacity may fluctuate as with some forms of mental illness. The fact that a person is terminally ill does not necessarily mean that their loss of mental capacity is permanent.

People can become confused temporarily as a result of many illnesses such as dehydration, retention of urine, heart failure or respiratory failure, hypothermia, shock, or fever due to infection. Longer lasting or permanent loss of capacity can occur after head injury or stroke. With dementia, it is permanent and gradually worsening, although there may still occasionally, early on, be periods of lucidity.

A psychiatrist or neurologist may be needed to diagnose a disorder or disability of the mind or brain, based on specialist investigations. If improvement in mental capacity is expected, the decision about medical treatment should be deferred. Treatment must be provided which will keep the patients future options open as far possible. This is important when a person who is mentally competent loses their competence suddenly through accident or illness.

Part 2: Are they Capable of the Processes Involved in Making a Decision? Can they:

Understand and retain information?

Weigh it in the balance and make a choice?

Understand the implications of the decision?

Communicate their wishes?

Answers to these questions may be obvious, as in advanced dementia or unconsciousness, but there are many situations which require time to assess and are a matter of judgement.

Communication Difficulties

Every effort must be made to overcome communication difficulties. Electronic devices can enable the patient to use the slightest hearing or vision to take in information, and tiny movements, such as the blink of an eye, to indicate what they wish.

The patient's ability to make decisions must be maximised by every possible help[8]. A person is not to be regarded as unable to make a decision unless all practicable steps to help him to do so have been taken.

The definition of a lack of mental capacity relates to a particular decision at the time that decision is to be made—the matter in question.

The Right to Consent to or Refuse Medical Treatment

The Mental Capacity Act 2005 is mainly for adults living with long term learning disability, dementia or mental illness, and is to ensure that decisions taken on their behalf throughout their lives are in their best interests. A patient with diminished mental capacity must be involved as far as they are capable, at a time and in a way which maximises their mental capacity. This covers giving or refusing consent to screening and immunisation programmes, investigations, medication, dental and ophthalmic care, admission to hospital, control of fertility, and decisions about specific treatments such as psychiatric drug treatment, sedation or electroconvulsive therapy. A person should not be excluded from making any decision within their competence.

Because mental capacity may be lost in old age or terminal illness, end of life decisions may also come under the Mental Capacity Act. Adults who are mentally capable have the legal right to refuse or consent to medical treatment. Doctors are completely familiar with that right. The Advance Decision takes forward that right to refuse life sustaining medical treatment, to a time in the future when you may lack mental capacity. This right underpins the legal status of the Advance Decision.

When to write an Advance Decision?

Now—while you are well, do not leave it too late.

The stimulus for writing your Advance Decision might be the death of someone close to you, or hearing of someone who has lived on after a severe head injury or stroke, or other devastating illness, but not regained mental capacity. You may have friends or relatives who have dementia. Though early diagnosis may allow time to write an Advance Decision, organisational skills and motivation can be substantially lost at an early stage of dementia, often before the diagnosis is apparent or accepted.

My motivation to write my Advance Decision while still in good health came from the circumstances of my parents deaths - my mother dying from Alzheimer's, my father from a stroke.

If I have a heart attack or other life threatening accident or illness in which I lose mental capacity suddenly, I would want every effort to treat me and restore my mental capacity.

But if my mental capacity could not be recovered, If terminally ill I would want my family and doctors to accept my Advance Decision to refuse life sustaining treatment.

The Advance Decision I have written allows scope for thoughtful discussion, because the clinical situations I have described are not detailed but allow of a judgement as to whether or not the situation is sufficiently 'advanced', 'serious', or 'disabling'. My statement of values indicates what these words would mean for me, if I had irrecoverably lost mental capacity.

I did not include detailed instructions as I have no disease to which these could refer, but in any case I do not think detailed instructions are helpful (see pp. 87-91).

After diagnosis or during progression of illness.
Many people are spurred into writing an Advance Decision by being diagnosed with an illness which might eventually prove fatal, such as heart failure, respiratory failure, diabetes, motor neurone disease, Parkinson's, multiple sclerosis, HIV, cancer, or other progressive or degenerative illness. Mental capacity is retained until a late stage in these illnesses. It becomes possible to write detailed instructions because you have a specific diagnosis, but such instructions remain optional.

All these eventualities are covered by my Advance Decision because I have described clinical situations in general terms, and not tried to be specific.

With advancing disease you may reach a stage of disease so severe and disabling that you would prefer to be allowed to die rather than face what lies ahead. Sudden fatal illness such as a heart attack or respiratory arrest would be a release. You might want to write detailed instructions to refuse resuscitation. Perhaps a DNAR (Do Not Attempt to Resuscitate) agreement would be what you are really asking for. Before adding detailed instructions to your Advance Decision you need to discuss this with your doctor to ensure that you are receiving all appropriate help and palliative care for your illness.

There are many pros and cons of detailed instructions (see pp. 87-91). In general, I think they are to be avoided. So long as you write an Advance Decision without detailed instructions, you do not need the advice of your doctor.

Writing your Advance Decision

You can write a letter or a formal document, but it is best to use a form, because this is likely to be the format doctors and nurses expect to see and will therefore most readily accept.

For my own Advance Decision I used as a basis the official NHS form available on the internet.[9] It rather focuses on detailed instructions and is difficult to fill in. I have made changes based on my reading of the Mental Capacity Act and the Code of Practice.

I also reviewed guidance and Advance Decision forms produced by patients' associations and societies which aim to help patients with various diagnoses, and agencies relating to old age and dying. (See pp 80-86). I have acknowledged and referenced the improvements I have made as a result. My Advance Decision is on page 73-79 and there is a blank copy of the form at the end of the book and on the website *www.advancedecision.uk*.

Written or verbal?

If you cannot write, you can give your instructions verbally and ask another person to fill in the form and sign it on your behalf, in your presence and in the presence of witnesses.

Who is your Advance Decision addressed to?

The meaning of the word 'Family'

Throughout this book I have referred to 'family' in the context of discussions with doctors about an Advance Decision. It includes parents, offspring and siblings, marriage partners and civil partners, and other relatives. However, many people are closer to workmates, friends, partners, neighbours or carers. It is difficult to cover all these possibilities without being long winded, so I have used the word 'family' as shorthand.

There is space on the form for the names and addresses of the people you want to be involved. These are the people you should talk to about what you would want should you have lost mental capacity when dying.

If you appoint a welfare attorney and want your Advance decision followed, you should indicate this on your Advance Decision, and ask your welfare attorney to sign it, showing that they know of its existence and will follow it. (See pp 91-93).

What Cannot be Requested in an Advance Decision

There are certain requests that cannot be made in an Advance Decision. You cannot:

request not to receive ordinary nursing care which is required to maintain hygiene and keep you comfortable. This includes offering water and food;

request anything illegal, e.g. euthanasia or (currently) assisted dying;

insist the medical team carry out any particular treatment.

How often should it be reviewed?

An Advance Decision will continue to have legal standing and will always be taken account of in decision making.[4] Appropriate times for review would be: on the appointment of a welfare attorney; on making detailed instructions; if your health changes or if developments in treatment for your condition arise.[10] Additions or changes should be signed by you and initialled by witnesses.

Who Should Have a Copy?

Two family members or friends, your welfare attorney (if you have one) and your GP. Have one placed in your hospital notes if you have had hospital treatment. If you make detailed instructions your hospital consultant and other doctors and nurses on the clinical team should be aware of it and have access to a copy.

Hospitals and GPs are gradually introducing a marker on your notes or computerised file which signals an Advance Decision. However, at present, an Advance Decision is usually brought to the attention of medical staff by a patient's family. Therefore you may wish to carry a card in your wallet or wear a *Medic Alert* bracelet or pendant with the relevant information. *Medic Alert*[11] will keep a copy of your decision to be faxed (after verification of the doctor's identity) to any doctor who requests it. This will ensure that your Advance Decision can be known about even when your family are not around.

The Advance Decision

The Advance Decision includes:

Identifying information about you;

A description of the circumstances in which the decision is applicable, including a Statement of Values;

The decision itself - that you refuse life sustaining treatment;

Optional detailed instructions.

Information about you

State that you are of sound mind and not under duress when making your Advance Decision. Doctors will assume you had mental capacity when you wrote it, unless there is evidence to the contrary.

Include details of your name, address and date of birth. *You must be over 18 years of age.*

Sign the Advance Decision in the presence of two witnesses, and give their names and addresses. They should sign and date your Advance Decision in your presence and state that it was signed by you.

The Statement of Values

You should make a Statement of Values to outline the background and motivation for your Advance Decision[12] (see p.68).

The *background* for my Advance Decision comes from my parents, my own life and the deaths I have witnessed. The *motivation* for my Advance Decision comes from a wish to face death realistically and stoically, a fear of losing my mind, and an unwillingness to die without dignity and being remembered that way by my family. Your statement regarding background and motivation should be attached to your Advance Decision. (See p. 79, 129-130).

Your Statement of Values may also include:

Choices for personal care (see p.130);

Choices for your body after death (see p. 139-145);

Choices regarding your funeral ceremony (see p. 137).

These additional documents may be attached to your Advance Decision or given to your family separately.

Applicable Clinical Circumstances

Loss of Mental Capacity

The Advance Decision comes into effect only if you have lost mental capacity and cannot consent to or refuse treatment (see p. 60). You must be unable to take part in the decision in question at the time that decision has to be made. So the first clinical circumstance is that you have lost mental capacity.

Description of Clinical Circumstances:

The schedule given below is not specific but in broad terms describes circumstances you can envisage at some time in the future. It is used as guidance for health professionals in considering when a person might wish their Advance Decision to be followed[13]. The schedule is suitable for any Advance Decision.

Suppose as a result of accident or illness you are now unconscious and if you are to survive, you need life prolonging treatment. Only your doctors and family (helped by your Statement of Values and what you have said in the past), can decide if you would prefer to go on living or be allowed to die. Your Advance Decision empowers them to consider these alternatives.

In a sudden illness, or worsening of a long standing illness, what outcome can be expected from treatment? Can mental capacity be recovered? To what extent can your state of health be restored? In dementia, has the point has been reached when pleasure and meaning in life are gone, or were you still enjoying life? If you have a disease which is now in its terminal stages, have you reached the point where this is an opportunity to slip away, rather than continue to struggle?

There are many questions which you cannot answer if you have lost mental capacity. 'Advance Decisions are more likely to be helpful if they reflect values and motivations rather than specifying clinical conditions or interventions in detailed instructions, which are in any case unlikely exactly to match the situation.'[12]

Rather than specific and particular detailed instructions, 'It is helpful to include a comprehensive and qualified description of circumstances and treatments in all Advance Decisions'[14].

In the schedule clinical situations are broadly described by using words such as 'advanced', 'severe', 'increasing', or 'comparable'. The Statement of values indicates what these words would mean for you and what outcomes you would find intolerable.

The Schedule

'Advanced Alzheimer's disease or any other form of dementia.

Severe and lasting brain damage due to injury, stroke, or other cause.

Advanced degenerative disease of the nervous system.

Severe HIV AIDS or other immune deficiency.

Advanced cancer with secondary spread not responsive to treatment.

Severe and increasing disability due to terminal cardiac or respiratory disease.

Any other condition of comparable gravity.'

Two appropriately qualified doctors working independently of one another should agree that I am unlikely to regain mental capacity or to recover from this illness or impairment, even though treatment is available which may prolong my life.

The Decision

The decision brings together the clinical circumstances and the refusal of treatment:

69

'If at any time I am unable to participate in decisions regarding my medical care, and

two independent doctors (one a consultant) are of the opinion that I am unlikely to recover from illness or impairment,

Then in those circumstances my directions are as follows:

I am not to be subjected to any medical intervention or treatment aimed solely at prolonging or sustaining my life **even if this means my life is at risk.**

The end of the above statement is very important because the Mental Capacity Act states 'the Advance Decision is not applicable to life sustaining treatment unless it is 'verified by the patient to the effect that treatment should be withheld or withdrawn even though my life is at risk'.[2]

If it is decided that my Advance Decision should take effect please also institute a Do Not Attempt to Resuscitate agreement.

Any distressing symptoms, including any caused by inability to eat, drink or simply receive nutrition, are to be fully controlled by appropriate palliative care.

Pregnancy

If pregnancy is a possibility you may want to include the following statement. It is on the form to be deleted or initialled.

'If I am suffering from any of the conditions described in the section above and I am pregnant, I wish to receive medical treatment leading if possible to the safe delivery of my child. Once my child is safely delivered I wish to reinstate my wishes as set out in the rest of this document[15]'.

Persistent unconsciousness

Below is the statement I have made in my Advance Decision.

'If as a result of head injury or stroke or other illness I remain persistently unconscious I wish doctors and my family to discuss my situation before considering invasive life support such as PEG feeding or tracheostomy.

Even if partial recovery of mental capacity may be possible, I do not want to live on with permanent severe disability either mental or physical, which would be burdensome to myself and my family. In circumstances where this would be the likely outcome I refuse life sustaining treatment even though my life may be at risk as a result. I would prefer to be allowed to die'.

Only you can choose when writing your own Advance Decision, whether to include these words from my Advance Decision, or delete them and use your own words. It will depend on your age, your current state of health and your attitude to the possible outcomes: living on in a persistent vegetative state; surviving with disabilities or the possibility of recovery.

At a younger age the brain has huge powers of recovery, and the future holds out possibilities for repair (gene or stem cell therapy) or the enabling help of electronics and engineering (computers and bionics).

Personally, at the age of 68yrs I am prepared to forego these possibilities, to avoid the risk of passing the remainder of my life with lost or severely diminished mental capacity. I would not want my family to remember me in that way.

My statement is open to discussion, to be informed by specialist medical opinion at the time, and backed up by my Statement of Values.

The more prescriptive instruction below is suggested by Compassion in Dying.[15]

'I refuse life prolonging treatment in the event that I am persistently unconscious and have been so for at least 2 weeks and there is little or no prospect of recovery (in the opinion of two appropriately qualified doctors).'

Read the notes about persistent unconsciousness due to brain injury (see pp 47-48).

Advance Decision to Refuse Treatment

To my family, my doctors and everyone concerned: this Decision is made by me when I am of sound mind, well informed and after careful consideration. If in future I lose mental capacity, and am terminally ill, in the clinical circumstances described I refuse life sustaining treatment, even though my life will be at risk and my death may be hastened as a result.

My Name Hilary Page	Any distinguishing features in the event of unconsciousness
Address	Date of Birth
	Telephone Number(s)

Mental Capacity

Please do not assume I have lost capacity. Find out about my medical history from my family, GP or hospital notes. I might need help and time to communicate.

Legal status

If I have lost mental capacity please check the validity and applicability of this Advance Decision. It must be taken into account in decisions about my medical care. I have indicated clinical circumstances when, if I am terminally ill and have lost mental capacity, I refuse life sustaining treatment. This does not preclude basic care and comfort.

Statement of Values

Please read my Statement of Values which outlines the background and motivation for my Advance Decision. It indicates clinical situations which I would find intolerable. Talk to my family, to help consider whether I would wish to refuse life sustaining treatment.

Applicable clinical circumstances

Loss of Mental Capacity

I have become unable to participate effectively in decisions about my medical care through loss of mental capacity or unconsciousness and

Two independent doctors (one a consultant) are of the opinion that I am unlikely to recover from illness or impairment and

Terminal Illness

I suffer from one or more of the following:

Advanced Alzheimer's disease or any other form of dementia;

Severe and lasting brain damage due to injury, stroke, disease or other cause;

Advanced degenerative disease of the nervous system (e.g. motor neurone disease);

Severe immune deficiency (e.g. AIDS);

Advanced cancer with secondary dissemination not responsive to treatment;

Severe and increasing disability from terminal cardiac or respiratory disease;

Any other condition of comparable gravity.

*(Schedule taken from Notes for Guidance to NHS staff when assessing an Advance Decision)

My Decision

In the clinical circumstances described above,

I refuse any medical intervention or treatment aimed solely at prolonging or sustaining my life, even though my life may be at risk as a result.

If my Advance Decision should take effect, please institute a Do Not Attempt to Resuscitate (DNAR) agreement.

Any distressing symptoms (including any caused by lack of food) are to be fully controlled by appropriate analgesia or other treatment, even though that treatment may shorten my life.

Unconsciousness due to brain damage
If as a result of head injury or stroke or other illness I remain persistently unconscious, I wish doctors and my family to discuss my situation before considering invasive life support such as artificial feeding via PEG tube or ventilation via tracheostomy. Even if partial recovery of mental capacity may be possible, I do not want to live on with permanent severe disability either mental or physical, which would be burdensome to myself and my family. In circumstances where this would be the likely outcome I refuse life sustaining treatment, even though my life may be at risk as a result. I would prefer to be allowed to die.

Pregnancy (Applicable / ~~Non-Applicable~~)
If I am pregnant and suffering from any of the clinical circumstances described above I wish to receive medical treatment or procedures to sustain my life in the hope of safe delivery of my child. Once my child is delivered I wish to reinstate my wishes as set out in this document.

Organ Donation (Applicable / ~~Non-Applicable~~)
I have registered with the NHS Organ Donor register. After brain death I wish for life support necessary to maintain for a time the viability of any of my organs or tissues suitable for donation.

My Advance Decision to refuse life prolonging treatment is to be followed even if my life is at risk as a result.

My Signature   **Date of Signature**

Witness Statement

The maker of this Decision signed it in my presence. I do not know of any pressure brought on him/her to make such a Decision and I believe it was made by his/her own wish. I do not stand to gain from his/her death.

Witness	Signed
Name	Telephone Number(s)
Address	Date
Witness	Signed
Name	Telephone Number(s)
Address	Date

My General Practitioner is: (Name)

Address

Telephone

The name of my Welfare Attorney is:
(applicable / ~~non-applicable~~**)**

The following list identifies people who have a copy and with whom I have discussed this Advance Decision to Refuse Treatment. Their contact details are provided. Any of them may be informed in a situation where I require medical care but have lost mental capacity to take part in discussions and decisions about treatment.

Name	Relationship	Telephone Number

Statement of Values (Optional but recommended)

Here you should attach a Statement of Values in your own words, or a letter to your family.

Background and motivation for my Advance Decision.

The background to my Advance Decision includes the deaths I have witnessed as a doctor and a daughter and seeing the Advance Decision in action. The circumstances of my parents' deaths, my mother from Alzheimer's, and my father from stroke, persuaded me to write one now, while still in good health, and not to wait until I became ill.

My motivation to write an Advance Decision comes from a wish to face death realistically and stoically, a fear of losing my mind, and an unwillingness to die in indignity, being remembered that way by my family. I fear pain, and want my pain to be relieved, even if this appears to hasten my death. I fear artificial nutrition by nasogastric or PEG tube.

I want those around me to accept my death, to be kind, and to be spiritually aware. I know my family will care about me, and I trust them to carry out my wishes as far as possible. I hope someone I love will be there with me at the end.

I am indebted to the doctors and nurses and the other people who have contributed to my care during my life, and especially thank those who will care during these last days of my life.

Below I describe situations I would regard as intolerable. I would prefer to be allowed to die a natural death than to continue in such a situation:

Ongoing mental disability to the extent that I lack mental capacity and am unable to respond to the love of my family or the kindness of friends and helpers , and unable to find meaning and enjoyment in any activities. (I will be grateful for help with any activities, so long as I still have enough mental capacity to enjoy them)

Physical disability - weakness, breathlessness, lack of movement or coordination, sensory loss, or severe pain, to an extent that independent function is a struggle and I have become a burden to myself and others in even basic activities such as eating and drinking, reading or listening to books, going to the toilet, bathing, dressing, taking part in conversation.

Please see *What Choices Have I Made?* regarding what happens to my body after death, and my funeral. Note that I have registered with the NHS Organ Donation Registry.

.

Detailed Instructions
(Optional - delete as required below)

~~Applicable~~
~~See detailed instructions below.~~

Non -Applicable.
*This Advance Decision was made **without** detailed instructions.*

THE ADVANCE DECISION ON THE INTERNET

I have looked at a range of health related websites to see what guidance and forms are on offer. Postal and website addresses are among the references at the end of the chapter.

Alzheimer's Association and *Motor Neurone Disease (MND) Association* have useful websites for patients and their carers, which include guidance on writing an Advance Decision and a form to use. The *Multiple Sclerosis Association* has an excellent website but little guidance on the Advance Decision - for this it refers to the website of the MND Association.

The websites of *Parkinson's UK*, the *British Heart Foundation* the *British Lung Foundation*, and *Headway* (the association for help after severe head injury) are useful for patients but provide little guidance on the Advance Decision. Variously they refer to *The Patients Association, Age UK* and *Compassion in Dying*.

The *Patients Association* refers to *Age Concern* (which amalgamated with *Help the Aged* some time ago to form *Age UK*. *Age UK* itself provides information about the Advance Decision, but no form. For that they refer to *Alzheimer's Association*. The *National Council for Palliative Care* provide useful information and a form, but their presentation is strongly biased towards cancer.

The following notes describe what I found in more detail. You may find here information and advice relevant to your own circumstances, and wording which you wish to add to your Advance Decision. My Advance Decision form has been influenced as a result of my reading. I have acknowledged and referenced the sources.

Compassion in Dying

Compassion in Dying[15] is the sister organisation of Dignity in

Dying which has campaigned for the legalisation of assisted suicide. Compassion in Dying provide good guidance and a well designed form for writing your Advance Decision including a downloadable 'Notice of Advance Decision' card to fit in your wallet, and a useful checklist. The guidance recognises that the needs of those who are in good health, or in the early stages of disease, but mainly fear loss of mental capacity, are different from the needs of people in the advanced stages of progressive disease, who will probably retain mental capacity but hope fear indignity, disability and suffering as their illness gets worse.

I might have used this form but for two things:

The legalistic introductory statement overplays the possibility of criminal action against a doctor: 'to treat the person named below contrary to the clearly expressed Advance Decision is likely to be civil trespass and/or a criminal assault.' It is not normal in seeking professional help to threaten with the law from the outset. Trust is required on both sides. In my own Advance Decision I make reference to its legal status only to show confidence that doctors understand my legal right to consent or refuse consent to treatment in this way.

My other reservation about this form is the instruction given about persistent unconsciousness: it is too prescriptive for me. This is a very personal choice (see pp. 47-49, 75).

Alzheimer's Society[16]

The guidance is aimed at people who have already been diagnosed with dementia. It does not include any schedule indicating a wider range of circumstances. There is space on the form for detailed instructions, thus:

'Please insert your personal requests here in relation to the types of medical intervention you would find unacceptable (for example, artificial resuscitation and/or an artificial feeding tube inserted through the stomach wall)'.

With the modern approach to early diagnosis of dementia, a person may remain articulate and purposeful for a time, and able to write an Advance Decision. However I think it would be a mistake to write detailed instructions at this early stage of dementia. It could be a despairing reaction to the diagnosis.

If an intervening illness such as heart disease or pneumonia, or an accident, should threaten to be fatal, it may be that with treatment an outcome could still be expected which would give further enjoyable and meaningful life.

In dementia mental capacity is lost as the disease progresses. By the time dementia has progressed to the stage when you might wish to make detailed instructions, it is unlikely you will still be mentally capable.

Alzheimer's Society[16] sensibly states 'It is up to you to decide how detailed you want your Advance Decision to be'. If you write your Advance Decision while you are well, without detailed instructions, you can use the schedule (see p. 68-69) which gives scope for your family to think about what you would want, supported by your Statement of Values.

It is a pity Alzheimer's do not give more explicit encouragement to write an Advance Decision while still in good health, without detailed instructions but with an attached Statement of Values. Dementia is the condition people most fear when they think about losing mental capacity towards the end of life.

Debilitating Neurological Degenerative Disease
Examples are:

Motor Neurone Disease

Multiple Sclerosis

Parkinson's Disease

These diseases can exist in mild forms and the symptoms of them can be treated. For many, life can go on for years without severe disability and the patient may well eventually die from some other disease. Mental Capacity is often retained until close to death.

The Motor Neurone Disease Association[17]

The form on the website[17] is based on the assumption that you have MND and have now reached a stage where you would prefer to die, should the issue of life prolonging treatment arise. The following thoughtful statement is suggested on the form:

'I am becoming progressively weaker and more disabled. This condition now causes great problems with daily activities including eating and drinking. I have talked about my feelings with my family. This is the right time for me to make this decision as I know MND is terminal and I wish to make choices about the way I die.

I wish to refuse the following treatments.....in these circumstances:

Cardiopulmonary resuscitation (restarting my heart/breathing ....in the event that I have a cardiac or respiratory arrest.

Assisted ventilation......if I can no longer breathe by myself without the help of a machine, or after simple attempts to help have been tried to position me, clear my airway and remove secretion.

Artificial feeding (via a tube in my stomach/drip) ...... when my motor neurone disease has deteriorated to the point that I cannot swallow safely, even with the help of others.

In May 2014 the MND association issued new guidance on planning for the end of life[18] (see p.46). They now consider a DNAR agreement more appropriate than the Advance Decision for refusal of cardiopulmonary resuscitation in cardiac arrest.

Multiple Sclerosis Society UK[19]

The MS society does not provide a form for an Advance Decision on its website.[19] Their booklet 'Support and Planning Ahead' provides detailed information about cardiopulmonary resuscitation, life support machines (ventilatory support) and artificial feeding tubes (PEG) tubes. The MS Society stresses the advantages of life prolonging treatment: artificial hydration and nutrition will make you feel better, as will assisted ventilation. They advise caution about refusing antibiotics and CPR. This positive approach is appropriate because MS mostly begins at a young age (20-40 years), its course is fluctuating, and does not inevitably progress. The form (see p. 190) would be suitable for a person wanting to write an Advance Decision after a diagnosis of MS.

For a situation where the disease has progressed to a stage of profound disability, if you want to make detailed instructions, the MS Society refers to the MND website, suggesting that the same wording for detailed instructions would be appropriate.

Parkinson's UK[20]

The Parkinson's Disease website does not provide a form for an Advance Decision. Their booklet 'Preparing for end of life: a practical and emotional guide' does not give an example of detailed instructions, but suggests that you consider:

Would you want the use of antibiotics in severe bacterial infection?
Would you want a drip if you were unable to swallow?
Would you want to be artificially fed?
What should happen if your heart beat or breathing stopped?
Would you like to be told by doctors how serious your condition is or would you prefer not to know?
Should your care concentrate on providing comfort and peace?'

These are very good questions to discuss with your family before writing an Advance Decision. Rather than using them as a basis for detailed instructions they can be covered in your Statement of Values. Then an Advance Decision without detailed instructions, (see p.190, www.advancedecision.uk) will enable your family and doctors to make the right decision for you if you lose mental capacity.

British Heart Foundation[21] and British Lung Foundation[22]

There is no form on either website. The BHF suggests: 'If you want to make a legally binding decision to refuse certain treatment, you can get advice on how to do this from a healthcare professional who knows your medical history'. The BLF has a paragraph headed 'Advance directive' which includes: 'you can leave instructions about whether you want to be rescuscitated if your heart stops, receive artificial ventilation in intensive care or whether to donate an organ after death.'·

If heart or lung disease progresses and the severity of pain, breathlessness, cough and disability have become so difficult that in another crisis you want to be allowed to die, detailed instructions refusing resuscitation in relation to cardiac or respiratory failure can be added to your Advance Decision. But rather than writing detailed instructions in an Advance Decision, I would suggest that you might more honestly request a DNAR agreement with the people looking after you, especially if you would prefer to die at home rather than be admitted to hospital (see p.118).

Headway[23] (Head Injury Charity)

In looking for information about the Advance Decision on this website I came across the *House of Lords Select Committee report on the Mental Capacity Act*[24]. The report recommends work to raise awareness among professionals and the general public of Advance Decisions, in order to allow people an opportunity to make treatment decisions themselves if they lose capacity in future perhaps after a devastating head injury. Clearly Headway are supportive of writing an Advance Decision while you are well. I hope that this report there will prompt a change in the presentation of the Advance Decision, with less emphasis on legalistic detailed instructions. More emphasis should be placed on the Statement of Values and the need for discussion based on a broad schedule of circumstances in which a person might prefer to refuse life prolonging treatment.

The National Council for Palliative Care[25]

As part of their Guide for health and social care professionals the website of the NCPC provides a form suitable only for people who want to write detailed instructions. This is suitable for people who have not hitherto made an Advance Decision and now are being helped by a health care professional at the end of life, in a palliative care situation, typically when dying of cancer. This reflects the high level of professional care for people dying of cancer and the fact that mental capacity is usually retained until the end or close to the end.

Any Advance Decision is effectively a plea for palliative care. The NCPC stress that no Advance Decision should be ignored, but it is a pity their website does not make it clear that any adult can write an Advance Decision, when they are well, or if they become ill, with any disease, not only cancer, so long as they have mental capacity.

Age UK [26]

Age UK (the amalgamation of Age Concern and Help the Aged) provide useful guidance on their website, but no form. They refer to the Alzheimer's Society (see p.81).

Patients Association.[27]

The Patients' Association has a section on 'Living wills: how to ensure your wishes are known when you can no longer make yourself understood'. The 'draft living will form' is not included in the pdf download. Readers are referred to Age Concern, from where they will find their way to Alzheimer's Society.

SHOULD AN ADVANCE DECISION INCLUDE DETAILED INSTRUCTIONS?

The emphasis on detailed instructions in much of the advice about Advance Decisions undermined my confidence in writing an Advance Decision while in good health. I have no diagnosis on which to base detailed instructions. Reading more widely, I discovered that Detailed Instructions, far from being necessary to an Advance Decision, can in fact be disadvantageous.

The positive influence of detailed instructions is that you will have sought information about your disease and had a heart to heart with your family and doctors. Open discussion will provide a better understanding about your wishes and form the basis for a Statement of Values, which will be more useful than detailed instructions in an uncertain clinical situation in the future.

Detailed Instructions and the legal standing of the Advance Decision

All Advance Decisions have legal status. Doctors know that it is *your legal right to refuse consent to treatment*, including to refuse life sustaining treatment in an Advance Decision. They are professionally motivated to give due regard to your Advance Decision, in good faith.

If sanctions against doctors are needed sufficient already exist through the hospital complaints procedure, the GMC and the Court of Protection (see p. 94). A doctor not giving due weight to any Advance Decision can be sued for negligence and their licence to practice withdrawn by the GMC[4,5]. The GMC can prevent them from working as a doctor in the NHS and privately. A civil action can result in compensation to the patient or their family.

The only difference with detailed instructions is: *'A doctor can be sued for criminal assault if the doctor was satisfied that the Advance Decision was valid and clinically applicable yet, in specific clinical circumstances described in detailed instructions, went on to give the specific treatment (also described in detailed instructions), to which consent was refused in those specific circumstances*[2].

So a doctor not immediately following detailed instructions could find themselves in the criminal court for keeping you alive. This is unlikely. A doctor acting in good faith, if in any doubt, before allowing a person to die, would discuss detailed instructions with medical and legal colleagues and with the patients family, and in any dispute seek the advice of the Court of Protection.

Unintended Death by Detailed Instructions?
Detailed instructions are applicable only if they reflect the clinical situation, but since they are 'legally binding' you may think doctors, fearing they could be sued for keeping you alive, might let you die when you had not intended it. This risk is more theoretical than real, but is the reason put forward to justify the need to seek the help of a doctor or lawyer in writing your Advance Decision. There are many safeguards in the Mental Capacity Act[2] and the Code of Practice[7] which indicate the primacy of the right to life. A doctor must be satisfied that the Advance Decision is valid and clinically applicable.

The Advance Decision will not be valid if the patient has said or done anything which seems to contrary to it, or if circumstances now exist which the patient seems not to have foreseen[2].

While the applicability of the Advance Decision is being assessed, doctors must[5]:

Start necessary treatment which is considered to be of benefit while the patient's *mental capacity* is determined.

Consider whether the patient is in the *end stage of a disease*, and whether death is expected within hours or days or over a longer duration.

Evaluate the *possibilities for treatment* and the likely benefits, burdens and risks of treatment.

The Mental Capacity Act Code of Practice states : 'nothing in an apparent Advance Decision stops a person providing life sustaining treatment or doing any act he reasonably believes to be necessary to prevent a serious deterioration in the patient's condition while a decision as respects any issue is sought.'[7]

Do you want a 'Do Not Attempt to Resuscitate' agreement?

You may write detailed instructions refusing cardiopulmonary resuscitation. But if you have a cardiac arrest, reading your Advance Decision will not be the doctor's priority. Resuscitation will come first. Unless doctors treating you in an emergency already know about your detailed instructions refusing cardiopulmonary resuscitation, an immediate clinical decision to withhold resuscitation is reserved for a DNAR agreement (See Chapter Five). The MND Association have recently (May 2014) changed their guidance on cardiopulmonary resuscitation,[18] advising that a DNAR agreement is a more appropriate way of refusing resuscitation.

Do detailed instructions help doctors?

Detailed instructions help lawyers because they provide a means of testing in court whether a criminal assault has occurred. Detailed instructions are very clear. They prohibit specific named treatments in specific circumstances.

Doctors may immediately recognise that detailed instructions fall wide of the mark when a decision regarding life sustaining treatment must be made. It is difficult when writing an Advance Decision to predict specific clinical situations which might apply in future. The actual situation will inevitably be more complicated or perhaps not covered by the detailed instructions.

Do detailed instructions reduce scope for clinical judgement?
For any Advance Decision doctors must diagnose your clinical circumstances including mental capacity, and consider treatment options and possible outcomes. The implied legal threat when detailed instructions are used undermines trust and can be a distraction: '*A less prescriptive Advance Decision without detailed instructions is less legally enforceable but allows scope for consideration of many factors. Paradoxically it is more likely to be followed in the spirit of the patient's wishes than one which may cause doctors to concentrate on legal aspects because they wish to avoid liability. Discussion between doctors and the patient's family or representative can focus on what the patient would want.*'[12]

Learning about you as a person from your family and reading your Statement of Values they must decide whether or not you would consent to the treatment they offer.

Alzheimer's Society[16] sensibly states 'It is up to you to decide how detailed you want your Advance Decision to be'. Parkinson's Society[20] says 'not every situation can be planned for in an Advance Decision'.

Are Detailed Instructions restrictive?
In the absence of a broader schedule, detailed instructions may be taken to be exclusive of other circumstances and therefore reduce the applicability of an Advance Decision. If your Advance Decision includes a wider schedule[13], as my own does, doctors need not be preoccupied with trying to fit your detailed instructions to the clinical situation in hand. They can use the wider schedule and your Statement of Values to support their decision making.
'*Refusals, and the circumstances in which they apply, can only be properly understood in the context of information that gives rationale and balance to these decisions. In this way the intentions behind*

the Advance Decision can be used to interpret the refusal more accurately.[14]

Do you want better palliative care?

Detailed instructions could be a cry for help or a plea for better palliative care; an early despairing reaction to bad news of diagnosis or treatment failure. Depression can give rise to a negative outlook. It is helpful to discuss your situation with your doctor so that you understand the implications of detailed instructions but more importantly so that your doctor understands how you are feeling and can get specialist palliative care help for your illness. Depression can be treated; there are many treatment options for symptoms of disease. Remember, palliative care is not only pain relief but also a series of different life-affirming interventions based on your needs and your family's needs (see p.31).

LASTING POWER OF ATTORNEY (LPA)

The Mental Capacity Act[2] introduced the 'Lasting Power of Attorney'. You can grant this power when you have mental capacity, to another person who then has the legal authority to make decisions on your behalf if you become mentally incapacitated. There are two types of Lasting Power of Attorney (LPA), one which covers property and affairs, the other covering personal welfare. As implied by the 'lasting' in the title, these powers have long duration and far reaching application. The arrangements for appointing and registering an LPA ensure that this legal power is granted to a responsible individual.[28]

The LPA (Property and Affairs)

If you have already given someone the Enduring Power of Attorney, this will still stand. The new Lasting Power of Attorney (Property and Affairs) covers financial affairs - decisions about education, employment, housing, pension and investment. The Power of Attorney must be registered with the Office of the Public Guardian(OPG), (part of the Court of Protection), before it can be used to gain access to the sources of income or the bank accounts of another individual who lacks mental capacity. While awaiting registration their affairs will be temporarily managed by the Court.

Social Services can apply to the Court of Protection to appoint a deputy, to make decisions for an individual who lacks mental capacity and has not made a Lasting Power of Attorney.

The LPA (Personal Welfare)

The 'welfare attorney' makes decisions regarding health, welfare, medical treatment and care, which the patient lacks capacity to make for themselves. The welfare attorney will give or refuse consent to medical treatment. There is a section on the form which applies to life sustaining treatment. If you include this section, doctors will refer to your welfare attorney for consent for this. A *previously written* Advance Decision is no longer applicable. If you write an Advance Decision *after* appointing a welfare attorney, the Lasting Power of Attorney is revoked unless you ask your Attorney to sign it, to the effect that they will follow it.

Should you appoint a Welfare Attorney?

I have not appointed a welfare attorney. For most people appointing a welfare attorney is a beaurocratic and expensive way of dealing with decision making at the end of life. Ministers agreed an overhaul was needed[24]. After a review the the system is now more user friendly[28].

Although guidance states that a welfare attorney must be registered with the OPG, doctors cannot wait for this to happen, they must do their best for the patient and this will include listening to the person you have chosen, whether as welfare attorney or named in your Advance Decision, or both. (A Lasting Power of Attorney must be registered with the Court before legal action can be taken with regard to any disagreement or complaint about medical treatment brought by the welfare attorney.)

You do not need a welfare attorney because unlike access to finance, health services are provided on the basis of need and cannot be denied or delayed when a patient is severely ill or dying. Doctors respect your right to give or refuse consent to treatment. They welcome an Advance Decision and the involvement of the family (or indeed a welfare attorney) when someone lacks mental capacity and is seriously ill. They want to know what would be the patient's wishes before deciding on life sustaining treatment.

When Can It Be Sensible to Appoint a Welfare Attorney?

Regarding end of life decisions, doctors assume that it is appropriate to talk to close family. The family may claim that a friend named in your Advance Decision is not an appropriate person to take part in discussions about your medical treatment. They could not make this claim if that friend was your welfare attorney, whose suitability would have been checked in the appointment process.

A welfare attorney might therefore be useful if a person does not trust members of their family to agree regarding medical care. Some people have families who hold different religious or moral views which might prevent them from fully representing the patient's wishes.

You may outlive members of your family and close friends, and in the end no-one is there to discuss your Advance Decision with doctors. If you think this might happen, you may feel more secure if you appoint a welfare attorney. It is easier for someone to be given this power by you while you are still mentally capable, than for them to obtain it later if you have lost mental capacity.

How Do I Appoint a Lasting Power of Attorney (Personal Welfare)?

Guidance on appointing a Personal Welfare LPA is available from the Office of the Public Guardian in the form of a free leaflet which can be ordered by post or seen online.[28] There is a 12 page form to fill in (though not every section will necessarily have to be completed), with 44 pages of guidance notes to help you. You need a certificate, from your GP, or solicitor to show that you are mentally capable and understand the powers you are conferring on your attorney. There is a 16 page guide for certificate providers and witnesses, who may or may not require a fee for their services.

The LPA cannot be used until it is registered with the Office of the Public Guardian—this costs £120. (But see pp. 93-94).

Doctors are likely to accept a welfare attorney as your representative, but the LPA must be registered before your welfare attorney can go to court in a disagreement. Then there would be a cost of £400 for the work required to bring the issue to Court and £500 for a hearing before the Court. Check the most recent fees on the website. There are exemptions or reductions for those in receipt of benefit.

You probably do not need to appoint a Welfare Attorney. Simply name in your Advance Decision the person(s) doctors should speak to. Make sure they have a copy of your Advance Decision and that you have discussed your wishes with them.

The Role of the Court of Protection.
The court is there to serve the best interests of those who lack mental capacity. The main involvement of the court is in decisions relating to property and affairs.

The court is able to convene quickly in order to resolve any urgent question. If there is no LPA, the Court itself may give or refuse consent to treatment, or appoint a deputy, to make decisions on the patient's behalf. The Court can also adjudicate on the existence, validity or applicability of an Advance Decision, but is not able to override a valid and applicable Advance Decision.

Doctors are advised to apply to the court in any disagreement with the patient's family, deputy or welfare attorney about medical decision making. Solicitors may also apply to the court if they are asked to represent anyone who feels others are acting contrary to an apparently valid and applicable Advance Decision.

Some medical decisions are so serious that an application must be made to the Court. These include decisions about withdrawing established (PEG) artificial nutrition and hydration, or switching off ventilation from patients in a persistent vegetative state.

CONCLUSION

There should be a change in the presentation of the Advance Decision, with less emphasis on detailed instructions and 'legally binding' and more emphasis on the personal Statement of Values. There are circumstances in which it might be a person's wish to be allowed to die rather than receive life sustaining treatment. It is the legal right of an adult with mental capacity to refuse treatment in these circumstances. I hope people will be encouraged to write an Advance Decision while they are well, to carry forward that right into the future when they may be terminally ill and have lost mental capacity. They can do this in an Advance Decision without any input from a doctor or a lawyer. The most important thing is to discuss your wishes and fears with your family. It is helpful to inform your Advance Decision by adding a Statement of Values.

REFERENCES

1. John Dryden (1631-1700) *Palamon and Arcite* Bk. 3.

2. *The Mental Capacity Act.* Office of Public Sector Information (Legislation) The National Archives 2005.

3. *Living wills: advance decision or directive.* Government, citizens and rights. Website: direct.gov.uk April 2010.

4. *Consent: Patients and Doctors Making Decisions Together. Guidance for Doctors.* General Medical Council 2008.

5. *Treatment and care towards the end of life: good practice in decision making.* Guidance for Doctors. General Medical Council 2010.

6. *Decisions relating to Cardiopulmonary Resuscitation.* British Medical Association, Resuscitation Council UK and Royal College of Nursing. BMJ Publications 2007.

7. The Lord Chancellor. *The Mental Capacity Act Code of Practice* Department of Constitutional Affairs April 2007.

8. *Assessment of mental capacity. Guidance for Doctors and Lawyers.* The British Medical Association and The Law Society. BMJ Books London 2007 (2nd Edition).

9. Sample form: *Advance Decision to Refuse Treatment: NHS Guide.* Website: adrtnhs.co.uk ('downloads') 2010.

10. *Advance Decision and proxy decision making in medical treatment and research.* BMA Ethics Committee 2009.

11. *The Medic Alert Foundation* 327-329 Tel: 0800 581 420. Website medicalert.org.uk 2014.

12. Bonner S, Tremlett M, Bell D. *Are Advance Directives legally binding or simply the starting point for discussion on patients' best interests?* British Medical Journal 2009; 339:b4667.

13. Clinical Policy Document C.026. *Guidance on Advance Decision to Refuse Treatment.* NHS Darlington Oct 2008.

14. Martin J, Swallow L. *A critique of the NHSADRT proforma.* British Medical Journal (Supportive and Palliative Care) 2011;1:103

15. *Guidance notes and form for an Advance Decision.* Compassion in Dying 2014. 181 Oxford Street London W1D 2JT. Tel 0800 999 2434 Website: compassionindying.org.uk

16. *Advance Decisions. Explanatory information and form. Factsheet 463.* Alzheimer's Society 2013. Devon House, 58 St Katharine's Way London E1W 1LB. Tel 020 7423 3500. Website Alzheimer's.org.uk

17. *Advance Decision to refuse treatment.* Information sheet No.19. Motor Neurone Disease Association 2014. PO Box 246 Northampton NN1 2PR Tel 08457 626262. Website: mndassociation.org

18. *End of Life: a guide for people with motor neurone disease.* Motor Neurone Disease Association May 2014.

19. *Support and Planning Ahead - for people severely affected by MS. MS Essentials No.16.* Multiple Sclerosis Society 2011. *372 Edgeware Road London NW2 6ND. Tel 020 8438 0700. Website: mssociety.org.uk*

20. *Preparing for end of life: a practical and emotional guide. Parkinson's Disease Association 2012. Parkinson's UK 215 Vauxhall Bridge Road London SW1V 1EJ Tel. 020 7931 8080. Website: parkinsons.org.uk*

21. *Why we need to talk about death and dying.* British Heart Foundation 2012. BHF Greater London House, 180 Hampstead Road, London NW1 7AW. Tel 020 138 6556 Website: bhf.org.uk

22. British Lung Foundation 73-75 Goswell Road, London EC1V 7ER Tel. 0207 688 5555 Website: blf.org.uk

23. Headway. Bradbury House 190 Bagnall Road Old Basford Nottingham NG6 8SF. Tel. 0115 924 0800 Website: headway.org.uk.

24. *The Mental Capacity Act. How well is it working? House of Lords Select Committee Report May 2014.*

25. *Advance decisions to refuse treatment: A guide for health and social care professionals.* National Council for Palliative Care 2010. The Fitzpatrick Building 188-194 York Way London N7 9AS. Website: ncpc.org.uk.

26. *Making a Lasting Power of Attorney. LPA Creation Pack – Personal Welfare. A guide for people who want to make a new LPA.* Office of the Public Guardian 2007. Archway Tower, 2 Junction Road, London, N19 5SZ. Tel:0845 330 2900.

27. Patients Association. PO Box 935 Harrow Middlesex HA1 3YJTel. 0208 423 9111. Website: patients-association.com.

28. Kenneth Clarke. *Annual Report of the Public Guardian Board.* Office of the Lord Chancellor and Secretary of State for Justice. 2012

29. *Advance decisions, advance statements and living wills.* Factsheet 72 Jan 2014. Age UK Tavis House, 1-6 Tavistock Square, London WC1H 9NA Tel. 0800 169 6565. Website: ageuk.org

Chapter 5

Do Not Attempt to Resuscitate?

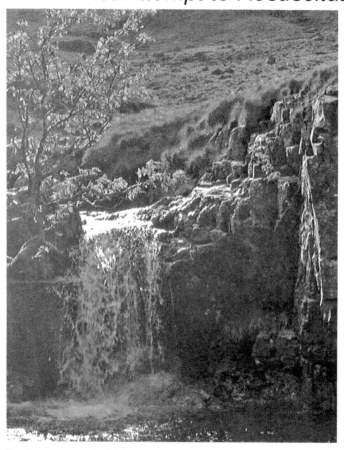

Gods, my gods! How sad the evening earth!
How mysterious the mists over the swamps!
He who has suffered much before death, bearing
on himself too heavy a burden, knows it. With a
light heart he gives himself into the hands of death,
knowing that she alone can give him peace."

Mikhail Bulgakov (1891-1940)

WHAT IS RESUSCITATION?

In Chapter Two causes of sudden death in terminal illness were described: heart attack, choking, pulmonary embolism, stroke, haemorrhage. Consciousness is lost because there is insufficient blood supply to the brain.

In any of these events an attempt may be made to restore consciousness by restoring the heartbeat and breathing - cardiopulmonary resuscitation.

Cardiopulmonary Resuscitation (CPR)

Cardiopulmonary resuscitation supports the vital functions of the body: the heartbeat and breathing. It is the combination of mouth to mouth respiration (the 'kiss of life'), and external cardiac massage (chest compressions which squeeze the heart to maintain the circulation). This first aid can be started immediately when a person has stopped breathing and their heart has stopped beating, and is followed as soon as possible by more technical support.

Cardiac Defibrillation

The patient may require cardiac defibrillation which you have seen on television programmes like Casualty and Holby City. (These programmes give an unrealistic impression of how successful CPR can be![2]) Electrodes are applied to the chest, everyone stands clear and a controlled electric shock is passed across the heart to make it start beating normally again.

Drugs, Drips, Masks and Tubes

Emergency resuscitation also involves injecting drugs and setting up an intravenous drip to help maintain the circulation. Oxygen by mask will also be used. In some emergencies, ventilation of the lungs is commenced by placing a tube through the mouth into the patient's windpipe (trachea).

Resuscitation can therefore be invasive. Some CPR attempts are traumatic, meaning that death occurs in a manner that the patient and those close to the patient would not have wished.[2]

Policy on Cardiopulmonary Resuscitation

When someone suddenly loses consciousness and their heartbeat and breathing have stopped, this is an emergency requiring immediate action. There is no opportunity to read a patients notes or talk to relatives. The British Medical Association, the Resuscitation Council UK, and the Royal College of Nursing in their joint statement 'Decisions relating to cardiopulmonary resuscitation'[3] say that unless there is a clear prior decision to the contrary, a Do Not Attempt to Resuscitate (DNAR) agreement, the best interests of patients are served by the immediate provision of CPR.

Successful Resuscitation?

In hospital, the chance of successful resuscitation and surviving to go home is only 20%. In a terminally ill or frail elderly person the chance of survival after resuscitation is particularly low. Complications such as fractured ribs, ruptured spleen or liver, can occur. Even 'successful' resuscitation is usually followed by a sojourn in intensive care with invasive ongoing life support which the patient may not survive.

There is also a risk that the patient will survive with brain damage, loss of mental capacity and disability. You can perhaps envisage a level of terminal illness and disability in which you might prefer to be allowed to die, without any attempt at resuscitation.

'The consequence of inappropriate resuscitation is an undignified death, distress to relatives, demoralisation of health care staff and poor use of resources'.[4]

Do Not Attempt to Resuscitate –Making an Agreement

The agreement not to resuscitate is relevant to the setting where the patient is, where everyone who will be on hand knows they must refrain from resuscitation if a cardiac or respiratory arrest occurs. 'Do not attempt to resuscitate' is not an agreement you can make when in good health, but when terminally ill and it is considered that a cardiac or respiratory arrest may occur. A patient can decide that if this happens, they would prefer to be allowed to die, rather than an attempt be made to resuscitate them[4].

Sudden unexpected cardiac or respiratory arrest may be the final event in any terminal illness, though it is most likely to occur in advanced cardiac or respiratory disease.

With terminally ill patients, doctors and nurses should sensitively initiate discussion about resuscitation. Sometimes a patient may initiate this discussion or provide cues, hoping that doctors or nurses will pick up on them. Discussion should be realistic about whether resuscitation could be successful and ensure that the patient is aware of their right to request that no attempt be made to resuscitate them. Some patients do not wish to discuss resuscitation or the possibility of a DNAR agreement.

If the patient has mental capacity there must be consent to any DNAR agreement. Where a patient has lost mental capacity, the Resuscitation Council guidance makes it clear that clinicians should consider and decide about resuscitation with those close to the patient.[3] An Advance Decision can help with deciding about a DNAR agreement.

Do Not Attempt to Resuscitate and the Advance Decision to Refuse Treatment

Neither doctors nor the patients family may override detailed instructions refusing cardiopulmonary resuscitation in an Advance Decision. It may therefore function like a DNAR but only if the doctor or nurse on duty knows about the Advance Decision and that it contains these detailed instructions.

An Advance Decision is a long and complicated document, possibly embedded in the notes, or perhaps just referred to, the main document being held by the family or the GP. The detailed instructions regarding cardiopulmonary resuscitation may have been written some time previously and may not cover the current clinical situation.

In contrast, the DNAR agreement is focussed and specific, and signalled by four capital letters on the patients notes. It is known to be current, having been recently discussed because the stage of disease has been reached that there is no wish for an attempt at resuscitation. This is not like an Advance Decision written for the future, it is a current agreement between doctors and the patient and/or those close to the patient if the patient lacks mental capacity. The settings where the patient might be are all covered:- in hospital or looked after in a nursing or residential home, or receiving care in their own home from their family or community nursing team. The people who might be present when a cardiac or respiratory arrest occurs are party to the agreement, and will refrain from any attempt at resuscitation[3].

Generally, in the absence of a DNAR agreement, it must be presumed that resuscitation would be in the patient's best interest.

Abandoning Cardiopulmonary Resuscitation
The general rule is that once someone has started CPR, other doctors and nurses coming on the scene should assist them, not start a debate about whether or not it is appropriate to attempt resuscitation in this case. If initial resuscitation has not been successful in maintaining the circulation and oxygen intake, or, if the patient is at the end stage of terminal of illness, a senior

clinician may decide that to continue the attempt at resuscitation would be invasive and burdensome beyond any possibility of benefit to the patient.[5]

During the process of CPR there may be the possibility of obtaining more information about the patient's previous state of health and what their wishes may have been. An Advance Decision, particularly if there are detailed instructions, may then lead to withdrawal of the resuscitation attempt.

Deciding to Withdraw Ongoing Life-Sustaining Treatment
In an emergency, unless there is a DNAR agreement, resuscitation will be attempted; and if the heartbeat can be restored, then ongoing life-sustaining treatment will be considered. The patient may recover mental capacity, and can then discuss the options with their doctors. For some people, if they are severely ill, this may be the opportunity to request a DNAR agreement.

The patient may remain unconscious or regain consciousness but with brain damage and loss of mental capacity. The doctors must decide whether or not to continue life-sustaining treatment. Stopping life-sustaining treatment is never easy. The advantage of the Advance Decision is that it opens the discussion, questioning whether further attempts to sustain life are what the patient would have wished.

Policy in Terminal Care Settings
It used to be that in some terminal care settings resuscitation would be discussed only if the patient asked. The policy was to refrain from CPR, on the basis that the patients were terminally ill. It is now considered that such a blanket policy would be unacceptable.[5]

Giving Patients the Opportunity to Decide
In hospices, on most hospital wards for elderly people, and in nursing homes, best practice is that patients with terminal illness

(or if not mentally capable, those close to them) are offered discussion about end of life topics[6]. If there is any likelihood of a sudden terminal event, a DNAR agreement should be discussed. This discussion will be raised when an appropriate opening occurs, after the patient has been assessed, and again later, as the clinical situation changes.[5]

(If the subject is not broached, it may be because there is little expectation of sudden cardiac or respiratory arrest occurring. A discussion about resuscitation and the possibility of a DNAR agreement would then be inappropriate and unkind. Doctors and nurses are under no obligation to discuss with patients every eventuality, however unlikely.[2])

An appropriate opening is more likely to occur if the patient has already discussed death with their family and written an Advance Decision.

Some patients (and perhaps some doctors) cope by being in denial and avoid such discussion. One writer has suggested that the phrase *"Do not attempt to resuscitate"* has an imperious and frightening ring to it. He suggested that perhaps it should be replaced by PEACE – Please End Attempts at CPR,[7] which more truly reflects the patient's wish to die in peace. Such a change in emphasis might make it easier to initiate discussion.

Training for Doctors and Nurses

Discussing a decision about resuscitation with a patient requires sensitivity, an awareness of the ethical issues involved, and clinical knowledge, all of which must be tailored to the needs of each patient, each person. There are widespread initiatives to provide a structured format for this discussion[8](see Chapter Six).

The National Audit Office[9] found that only 39% of doctors and 15% of nurses had received any preregistration training in communicating with patients approaching the end of their life. Specialised training had been received by 29% of doctors and 18% of nurses working in end of life care. Perhaps not all doctors and nurses have adequate training in end-of-life counselling, including discussion about resuscitation.

However, doctors and nurses think and read about these issues, learn from experience, talk to their colleagues, patients and patient's relatives. They are professionals who educate themselves in many ways – for example by reading and discussing the Report of the Resuscitation Council[3] which was summarised in the British Medical Journal[5]. Death and dying are becoming more widely discussed by everyone. We all have an interest.

DNAR at Home

When a patient is suddenly very ill they may be admitted to hospital even if death has been expected and the patient wants to die at home. If the community nursing services are not geared up to immediately providing help, the family and/or the care home staff would not find it acceptable to allow the patient to die at home, because the symptoms of pain, anxiety and breathlessness are very distressing. Without Advance Planning to cope with this crisis at home, the patient will be admitted to hospital.

Hospital doctors may have little information at first and must presume that the patient wants to go on living. They will attempt resuscitation and instigate life-sustaining treatment. The patient, who wished to die peacefully at home, may now suffer a more protracted death in hospital.

An Advance Decision and ultimately a DNAR can be used in Advance Planning (see pp. 124-128). This will enable a high level of community nursing support to be immediately provided in an emergency, to help with the distressing symptoms and allow a particular patient, who wishes it, to die at home.

REFERENCES

1. Mikhail Bulgakov (1891-1940). *The Master and Margarita.*

2. Bass M. *Should patients who are at the end of life be offered CPR?* Nursing Times 27 January 2009.

3. *Decisions Relating to Cardiopulmonary Resuscitation.* British Medical Association, Resuscitation Council UK and the Royal College of Nursing. BMJ Publications 2007.

4. *Resuscitation and your right to refuse it.* Website: direct. gov.uk 14 March 2009.

5. Conray SP, Luxton T, Dingwall R, Harwood R, Gladman JRF. *Cardiopulmonary Resuscitation in Continuing Care Settings.* British Medical Journal 2006; 332: 479-482.

6. Munday D, Pterova M, Dale J. *Exploring preferences for place of death with terminally ill patients: qualitative study of experiences of general practitioners and community nurses in England.* British Medical Journal 2009; 338; 214-217.

7. Crampton J. *DNR or PEACE?* British Medical Journal 2008; 336: 1015.

8. *End of Life Care.* National Audit Office. 2008 *A Programme for Community Palliative Care.* Royal College of General Practitioners and Gold Standards Framework

9. The NHS End of Life Care Programme. RCGP Publications 2008.

Chapter 6
The Choice of Where to Die

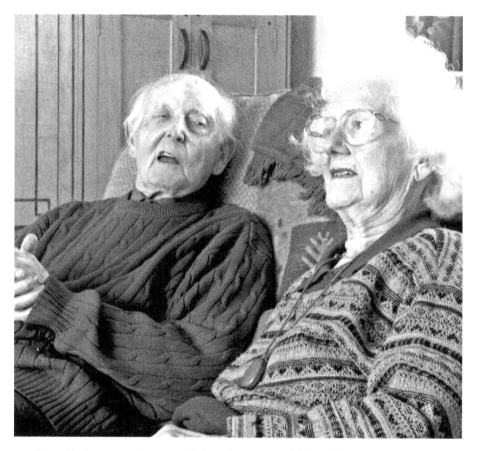

Death has got something to be said for it:
There's no need to get out of bed for it;
Wherever you may be,
They bring it to you, free.

Kingsley Amis (1922-1995)

Where do people die? And do most people get their preference for place of death? The answer to that question is: No.

Place of death for people aged over 75 yearsONS 2015[2]

	Men		Women	
	Number	**%**	**Number**	**%**
Hospital	86,151	60.8	108,736	55.0
Home	26,443	18.6	26,816	13.6
Nursing Home	13,598	9.6	29,666	15.0
Residential Home	8,963	6.3	25,643	12.9
Hospice	5,211	3.7	5,029	2.5
Other	1,309	0.9	1,554	0.8
All deaths aged over 75	**141,675**	**100**	**197,654**	**100**

DYING IN YOUR OWN HOME

Most people say they want to die in their own home.[3] This is much more likely to happen for people who still have their husband or wife living and able to look after them. Many more male deaths than female deaths occur at home simply because women live longer than men. Many men aged 75 years or over still have a wife who can look after them at home, if she is well enough.

Fifty percent of people aged over 75 years have a limiting illness or disability. Chronic but non-life-threatening conditions such as arthritis, osteoporosis, and loss of hearing and/or vision cause years of disability among the elderly. Added to these are dementia, circulatory disease, respiratory disease and stroke - the diseases which also cause the majority of deaths.

Women live longer, but they have more years of illness or disability than men.[4,5] The disability or illness of the spouse means that care of a dying person at home may be difficult. Many more people could die at home, if adequate social care and community nursing care could be provided. Even people who live alone can stay at home so long as they are mentally capable of organising their care as they become more frail. Progress has been made, but still the lack of community based services causes many to remain unnecessarily in hospital.

DYING IN A CARE HOME

Care homes include nursing homes and residential homes. Nursing Homes care for people who are physically very ill and need high levels of nursing. Some nursing homes specialise in the care of people dying from dementia. Residential homes are for those who are unable to continue to live at home through frailty, disability and the lack of support. 15.9% of men and 27.9% of women aged over 75 years die in care homes.[2] The difference in these percentages is large, but the actual number of women compared to men is even more striking (see Table 2) as there are so many more women over this age.

Many old people say *'Don't put me in a home,'* but in fact, especially for women, this wish is unrealistic. It stems, unfortunately, from a belief that care homes are worse than they really are, and prevents people from thinking about what care homes could and should be like. Newspapers and television seek out and publicise examples of cruelty and abuse - these do exist, and there have been shocking deficiencies in the system for inspecting and regulating care homes. Even so, the majority of care homes provide a homely setting and good care. When the time comes, people can die peacefully in the home where they live, close to their family and friends.

DYING IN HOSPITAL

What is the hospital for? Hospital doctors are trained to diagnose and cure disease, to defy and outwit death, not to go along with it. Many doctors are likely to interpret fatal signs and symptoms as a challenge to their clinical ingenuity. Most of the time this is what we want them to do, and this is why hospitals are equipped with all the modern technology of medicine – to save life.

Pressure on Hospital Care

Examples of recent problems with NHS hospitals are overcrowding of A&E departments and delay in admission for emergencies to an appropriate ward. Even in summer, some hospitals are forced to use surgical beds for acutely ill medical patients.

For an elderly person who has several disabilities and who is terminally ill, rather than admitting them to hospital, it may be more appropriate to allow them to die with comfort and dignity in their own home or a care home, where they live, if that is what they want.

The arrangements for getting people discharged from hospital or finding a suitable care home for them often take too long. People may die in hospital because they eventually succumb to hospital acquired infection or pulmonary embolism. Increased availability of care home places and community based palliative

114

care including emergency care would give people a choice of where to continue their lives, and a choice of where to die.

A doctor writing in the British Medical Journal described how her father's anxiety level rose every weekend and especially at bank holidays, fearing that 'if he should be taken ill he would be shunted off to hospital by the on-call services unfamiliar with his case and not knowing him as a person.'[6] This is exactly what happened. He was taken to hospital and subjected to investigations and invasive treatment, rather than being allowed to stay put and die quietly at home as he would have wished. Arriving later, his daughter was able to arrange his transfer to a nursing home near where they lived, where he received palliative care and died a few days later.

After reading this, another doctor wrote a letter describing how he had managed to get his dying father out of the acute hospital and into a place where the staff 'actively treated my father as a person, not as a complex medical puzzle'.[7]

Hospital Visiting

To many people a great drawback of being in hospital is the distance to be travelled from home by visitors and the constraints put on visiting times. Visiting often involves two bus journeys, or battling in a car with the traffic and having to find a car parking space at the hospital. The family, especially an elderly spouse, becomes exhausted. In winter, the cold and dark evenings add an element of risk, particularly for elderly people.

Privacy

A precious quality missing in hospital is privacy, to talk freely and be physically close to the person you love who is dying. This lack of privacy can cause the dying person to be isolated from the people they know and love.

Infections

Specific infections, to which frail elderly people are particularly susceptible, are much more likely to spread in hospital than in the community. *Methicillin Resistant Staphylococcus Aureus* (MRSA) can infect the skin or go deeper into an operation wound or pressure ulcer and cause blood poisoning. *Clostridium Difficile* causes stomach pains and severe diarrhoea which can be fatal in a person already frail.

Many frail elderly patients who die of these infections are, in any case, close to death, but if it were not for the infection, they could possibly have had a more peaceful death at home or in a care home. Instead of this they must undergo the hospital's efforts to treat the infection and prevent it spreading.

There has been a campaign in the NHS to improve hospital hygiene and other aspects of care in order to prevent these infections. The national monitoring of these infections shows that their incidence is falling[8,9,10] as a result of better cleaning, lower bed turnover and better hand washing facilities for visitors. Restriction of numbers of visitors and visiting hours also helps.

Poor Nutrition

Food is often impersonally served and sometimes there is little help to eat it. Elderly people in hospital are not always given the time or help they need to eat. Inadequate food intake may go unnoticed.[11] This is not likely to be a direct cause of death, but may weaken a person and delay their discharge from hospital, giving more opportunity for other problems to occur.

Pulmonary Embolism

Patients in hospital, if they cannot walk independently, may spend hours sitting beside their bed. Physiotherapy is provided, but this is typically for only half an hour a day. Visiting time, when a friend or relative walks up and down the hospital corridor with the patient, might be the only other time they leave their chair.

People confined to their bed, or sitting for long hours beside their bed in a chair, are prone to develop a clot in the vein of the leg - deep vein thrombosis (DVT). A piece of the clot can break off and travel in the bloodstream to the lungs, which may be fatal – a pulmonary embolism (see p. 17).

These problems are made much of by the media and contribute to the sense that the NHS is in constant danger of being overwhelmed, even though, in fact, a lot is being done to provide more services in the community and better links with social services. Also, so much more is offered by modern medicine for people who need to be there for medical reasons.[12]

DYING IN A HOSPICE

Hospices set the standard for palliative care for people dying from cancer, but in the over 75's only 5,211 (3.7%) of male deaths and 5,029 (2.5%) of female deaths occurred in a hospice.[2]

A huge increase in provision of new hospices would still only meet the needs of a small percentage of people. Therefore, when I support a campaign to increase hospice provision, I do this on the basis that many of our nursing homes should function more like hospices; and that ways must be found to bring hospice-type care (palliative care) into the places where people die[7]. The need for better palliative care for diseases other than cancer, and for old people, has only recently been recognised.[13] Palliative care must be extended on a much larger scale than at present: into hospitals, into care homes and into people's own homes.

CAUSES OF DEATH AND THE PLACE OF DEATH

The National Audit Office[3] found that the factors which influenced the place of death were age, geographical location and most significantly the cause of death. The disease determines the nature of the path from independent living to death – known as the 'trajectory' of a disease. The trajectories of different diseases are described in Chapter Two.

How Does the Trajectory of Disease Affect the Place of Death?

The loss of mental capacity, the extent of physical disability, the frequency of medical emergencies, the severity of symptoms and the ability to predict death all influence the possibility of providing care in different settings.[14]

For each of the main causes of death, I have summarised the trajectory and described how this influences the place of death. By doing this it becomes easier to understand how things could change to allow more people their choice of place of death, usually in their own home, or in a familiar care home in their neighbourhood, rather than in hospital.

Cancer - The Trajectory and the Place of Death

Diagnosis of cancer is often followed by immediate debilitating treatment – an operation, radiotherapy and/or chemotherapy which weakens the immune system and causes unpleasant side effects.

After this initial trauma there is a long period of 'living with cancer', often for several years with intermittent episodes of treatment, but otherwise feeling reasonably well and able to continue normal life without severe disability. Many are cured.

Eventually the cancer may spread out of control causing rapid decline. At this point death is predictable, and often likely to occur within a few months. Symptoms are controllable and the patient understands what is happening to them. It is therefore often feasible to die at home, with advice and support from specialised nursing services based in the hospice. If more complex care is needed, hospice care is available.

Cancer is the predominant cause of premature death between the ages of 45 and 74 years.[15] People who die from cancer often have a spouse or partner who is in reasonable health who can help to manage at home. The dying person usually remains mentally capable until close to the end. Also, the period of severe physical disability may be relatively short, the patient becoming bed bound only a few days before death. Therefore cancer is not a likely cause of being admitted to a care home.

The services for people dying at home from cancer are highly developed, based on the hospice model and supported by local hospices. Two famous nursing charities, Marie Curie Cancer Care and MacMillan Cancer Support, provide specialist home nursing services, linking with the community nursing team. The patient can be admitted to the hospice to give the carer a break, or for specialised medical care to bring a difficult symptom under control.

Those dying from cancer at any age are more likely to die at home than people of the same age dying from other diseases. If things are too difficult, the patient may be admitted to the local hospice within a day or two of death. Among hospice deaths the vast majority are from cancer, though only about 4% of all cancer deaths occur in a hospice.

Heart Disease and Chronic Respiratory Disease - The Trajectory and the Place of Death

Chronic heart disease and chronic respiratory disease both lead to long-standing disability which gradually increases and later gets worse after each life threatening emergency. Disability is from breathlessness, cough, chest pain and exhaustion. Death is unpredictable. Life is repeatedly saved and prolonged by hospital treatment. In the end the patient's life cannot be saved and they die in hospital – the most usual place of death from heart disease or respiratory disease.

Terminal heart or respiratory diseases now affect an older age group in which many live alone and with increasing disability.

They may move into a care home, often after a stay in hospital. Therefore, many people with severe chronic heart or respiratory disease live in care homes.

A person with chronic heart disease or respiratory disease who lives at home or in a care home may in the morning be too breathless to eat or take part in conversation, but still able to watch the birds or listen to visitors chatting, read a book or do the crossword. A couple of hours later they may be severely breathless, totally unable to speak and confused or even unconscious.

The possibility of being at home with someone you love dying in this way is frightening. The staff of a care home may be criticised if someone dies like this and is not admitted to hospital. The patient needs hospital treatment, unless immediate nursing support can be provided in a crisis, to control symptoms and support the family. Then the patient could die where they are most at ease, in their own home or familiar care home.

Sometimes the impetus for hospital admission comes from the relatives who want 'everything possible' to be done. They want to show their love for their parent and not to be the one who says 'perhaps we should let mother die, I think that is what she would want.' Another situation is where a relative who lives far away, comes to visit and cannot accept or tolerate the realisation that the parent is dying, and 'no one is doing anything about it.'

If the patient would prefer to die at home or in their care home next time there is a crisis, with detailed 'Advance Planning' (see p. 123) and the promise of immediate nursing support, it may be feasible to let them stay put and die peacefully. Advance Planning is usually initiated by the GP or community nurse. It includes an Advance Decision to Refuse Treatment, a Statement of Values and possibly a Do Not Attempt to Resuscitate agreement.

However, even when the intention is to manage death at home, anxiety, pain and breathlessness can be so severe and distressing, that the patient suffers too much and the family is overwhelmed. The Audit Commission accepted that one of the reasons people with heart or respiratory disease are more likely to die in hospital is that hospital support is sometimes needed to manage distressing and alarming symptoms, where the prognosis is uncertain.

Stroke - The Trajectory and the Place of Death

Death from stroke can be sudden and unexpected, but more commonly a person goes from being well, through transient ischemic attacks, to a minor stroke which leaves some residual disability. Further strokes will cause increasing disability. The person will eventually need support to continue living in their own home, or they may need to move into a care home.

Often after a severe stoke the patient is not mentally capable. Even if conscious they may have limited understanding or insight to weigh up decisions, and they may be unable to speak.

Admission to hospital will be needed to investigate the cause, the extent and the prognosis of the stroke. Hospital admission after stroke is therefore the norm and the majority who die from stroke die in hospital.

If there is an Advance Decision it will not be acted on in haste, but after allowing time for the patient's mental capacity and speech to improve. If mental capacity does not improve, and investigations show that it is unlikely to be restored, then the medical team will consider the Advance Decision. The medical team and family may agree that a DNAR agreement is also appropriate at this stage.

The patient may survive the stroke and later leave hospital to live at home or in a care home. A person who is already severely

121

disabled by previous strokes, might prefer to be allowed to die at home, or in their care home, if they have another stroke. The patient (or if they are not mentally capable, those close to them) may discuss a 'Do Not Attempt to Resuscitate' agreement with the carers and doctors.

Dying at home would be feasible only if the community nursing services, the general practitioner and the family were in agreement that they could be adequately nursed there. At present, except in health authority districts where services are highly geared to the needs of people dying at home, the patient is likely to require admission to a nursing home to cope with the heavy nursing demands.

The following scenario illustrates that hospital admission is not inevitable and that doctors are beginning to think more about the care of dying people at home.

A family did not understand that their mother had reached the end of the road.[16] She had previously had a stroke, and while in hospital she developed pressure sores and a chest infection. She vowed that she would not return to hospital should she fall ill again. She stated unequivocally that she would rather die at home. When the mother had another stroke, her husband had unrealistic expectations of what could be achieved. He called an ambulance to admit her to hospital and later insisted that she be artificially fed via a nasogastric tube and that she should be resuscitated if she had another stroke or a heart attack.

The doctor helped the family come to terms with her inevitable decline and death. The husband realised that invasive treatment was no longer humane. Palliative care at home was arranged to be provided by the GP and the community nursing services, with the daughter's help.

Dementia - The Trajectory and the Place of Death

A gradual onset and a slow decline characterise dementia. There is confusion, loss of memory, loss of emotional and behavioural control and self neglect. The majority die in a care home.

The course of dementia typically lasts about seven years. During most of this time the person can live at home, especially if they do not live alone. Sometimes it is possible for someone to continue for a time on their own - in sheltered accommodation or supported by a relative or friend living nearby. Familiar surroundings are important while the person is still aware and able to get about their home.

The impact of the illness is unpredictable. Unless sudden death from another cause intervenes, a person with progressive dementia is not likely to die at home, because the difficulty for the (usually elderly) spouse, or sometimes a daughter or son looking after them, is too great.

People with advanced dementia who can no longer be supported in their own home usually end their days in a nursing home specialising in the care of the Elderly Mentally Ill. Others die in hospital, having been admitted with another health problem - a fractured hip or chest infection, for example. People with dementia are difficult to care for in an acute hospital because they cannot understand what is happening to them or make their needs known. We need to increase knowledge, develop skills and change attitudes, in order to provide appropriate care for people with advanced dementia in hospital.

It is amazing to me what a devoted carer can do, especially if there is a supportive family. Unfortunately, the 'breaking points' for care at home (see p 29), do not coincide with the person's eventual loss of awareness of their surroundings, nor with their loss of ability to respond to love. When the breaking point comes, the demented person is removed from their familiar surroundings and from the person who loves them. This can be a source of great grief and guilt to carers. The aim should therefore be to provide small local nursing homes close to where people live, so that carers can visit easily.

The inexorable progress of dementia eventually destroys the swallowing reflex. A person with dementia may then be kept alive by artificial nutrition, in a nursing home. This is the most likely place of death for someone with dementia. The Advance Decision can allow the family or the patient's representative to suggest that artificial nutrition be withheld, and to initiate discussion about the aims of treatment. The patient can be allowed to die with their symptoms well controlled, careful nursing and sufficient hydration. Without an Advance Decision it is more difficult for the nursing home staff or the family to suggest the possibility of withholding artificial nutrition.

Frailty and Gradual Decline - Trajectory and the Place of Death
This is the process of gradual withdrawal, loss of appetite, weakness, forgetfulness and passivity, combined with the physical deterioration of old age, sensory loss, and multi-organ failure.

These old people often struggle on for several years, gradually declining and becoming more frail and dependent. If they have a husband or wife who is well enough to look after them, they may continue to live in their own home, and die there.

Some frail old people manage to live alone with informal help from family, friends and neighbours for many years. Gradually social services and community nursing services increase their input. Eventually this may break down, for example if the family go on holiday, or social services personnel are ill, or if the old person has a fall. The inevitable crisis may result in hospital admission. The old person may die in hospital, or survive and later be discharged from hospital into a care home. Frail old people often end their lives in a care home, but too many are admitted to hospital and die there.

Usually, however ill they are, it is possible to prolong a person's life by admitting them to hospital. Some frail elderly people who have severe disabilities and a poor quality of life might not want this, but are too ill to make the decision or to make their wishes known at the time. People suffering from the gradual decline of old age could be helped to stay put in their own home or a care home when they are dying, rather than be admitted to hospital.

The problem of too ready admission to hospital is discussed in medical journals. As a hospital consultant described, 'there is undignified death in hospital of those who simply have multiple pathologies related to ageing, and whose quality of life has deteriorated'.[17] He suggested that families and carers of elderly people in their own homes, or in care homes, should ask, 'If you become seriously ill again, what do you want us to do?' Then when another crisis occurs, the result is not automatic admission to hospital. This would prevent elderly very frail people from being 'over investigated or over treated because their circumstances were not adequately assessed in the community.'

ADVANCE PLANNING - MAKE 'STAYING PUT' FEASIBLE

Most people would prefer to die at home – so how can you plan for this? The NHS Strategy for End of Life Care[18] aims to make it possible for many more people to die at home.

The Preferred Place of Death

A study of place of death was carried out in Leigh, Lancashire.[19] Even when it was accepted that they were dying and would prefer to die at home, patients were admitted to hospital shortly before death. The main reason for this was that in the hours or days before death the patient and their family needed immediate support, and the NHS was not organised to provide that at home. The researchers gave the title to their study 'Place of death - Hobson's choice or patient's choice?'

Working with general practitioners and community nurses, they developed a local initiative called the 'preferred place of death.' This is an agreement between the patient (or if not mentally capable, their family) and those providing their care at home or in their care home. Close to death, increased nursing and other help is needed to make the patient comfortable, to relieve anxiety, and to support the family or care home staff. It is agreed that should a sudden worsening of the patient's condition occur, the community nursing service will immediately step up to meet the patient's and the family's increased needs. It is this agreement which makes 'staying put' feasible. This initiative enabled patients to have palliative care in their choice of place of death.

Doctors, nurses and social workers can plan with the patient, carers and family how to prevent hospital admission if the patient suddenly gets worse in the last weeks of life. Some local NHS services and nursing homes already work in this way, which is being encouraged by the many national initiatives described in Chapter One - in particular the Preferred Priorities for Care.[20]

The Advance Decision and Preferred Priorities for Care.

The ideas first developed for the 'preferred place of death' have evolved into a system of nursing in the community based on the patient's personal preferences and needs – the 'Preferred Priorities for Care' (PPC). This approach to nursing at the end of life is being encouraged within the NHS as an example of good practice which should be more widespread. Patients who want to die at home are helped to think about writing an Advance Decision to Refuse Treatment (if they have not already done so) and if appropriate a Do Not Attempt to Resuscitate agreement. The NHS provides training for doctors, nurses and other professionals so that they feel comfortable talking to patients and their families about these choices.

NICE Guidance for End of Life Care for Adults[21]

When death is imminent, palliative care to make the patient comfortable and support the family takes precedence over life-sustaining treatment.

Guidance produced by the National Institute for Health and Care Excellence describes a structured approach to the effective control of symptoms and the emotional support of the patient and their family. The guidance is to be used in all settings, home, care home, hospice and hospital. It brings together the many initiatives I have described in this book, and other examples of good practice. The guidance includes a section on information for the public, and is intended to involve the patient (as far as they are able) and the family in discussions about their needs, and about how to help the patient to have a good death.

The NICE Guidance covers aspects of service provision and treatment in palliative care, and describes standards which should be acheived in an excellent National Health and Social Services. NICE also provide measures by which the acheivement of these standards can be judged - the basis for reviews by the Care Quality Commission[22]. I think these Guidelines and Standards are useful, as a basis for improvement. They reflect the ideals of the work on 'a good death' (see p. 2-3) and the wide scope of the aims of palliative care (see pp 8, 31).

This approach will strengthen local collaboration between NHS hospital trusts and independent hospitals and hospices, care homes, GP practices and out of hours services, community services and home care agencies. The NHS and Local Authorities will be encouraged to provide balanced and joined up care.[18]

How your Statement of Values Can Help

If you have lost mental capacity, doctors and nurses must be guided by your family, as to your wishes about ongoing medical treatment, and preferences for personal care. It is very helpful if you write a Statement of Values (see p. 112) as well as an Advance Decision.

The Statement of Values can outline your preferences for your personal care; likes and dislikes for your environment, your clothing, hygiene and personal care, food and drink, music, and other aspects of life which are important to you.

Most importantly, a statement of values describes the background and motivation for your Advance Decision. Your Advance Decision allows doctors to decide to withhold or withdraw life sustaining treatment, without fear of being accused of ageism or of negligently allowing you to die when you could have been kept alive longer. Your Statement of Values will help them make this decision based on your wishes, when you are terminally ill and have lost mental capacity. Your Statement of Values gives detail and meaning to discussions between doctors and your family as to what your wishes would be.

You may name who you want to be involved in discussions about your care and who you want (or do not want) to see. You can describe what sort of religious or spiritual help you want. You can remind your family that you are registered with the NHS Organ Donor Register[23] and advise them about your body after death and about your funeral.

You can also use your Statement of Values to make clear your views about euthanasia and assisted dying. These are against the law in the UK. In future the law may change. An expression of your views might be helpful in either preventing or enabling assisted dying (if you have mental capacity) or euthanasia.

My own Statement of Values follows at the end of this chapter.

Take the Initiative

It is not up to doctors and nurses to prevent a dying patient going into hospital on the unspoken assumption that the patient would rather die at home. Doctors must assume everybody wants medical expertise directed towards saving their life. On clinical grounds they can withhold or withdraw treatment which would be unduly invasive and burdensome and without benefit to the patient, but they are not empowered to make a decision based on a judgement of the value of someone's life.

It is up to you to think about situations where they would prefer to be made comfortable and allowed to die in the natural course of events. Talk to your family, write an Advance Decision and a Statement of Values.

Meet the Care Providers Half Way

The Government, in developing NHS and Social Services policy, is receptive to the idea that more people should be enabled to die at home or in a care home in their own neighbourhood. If many people make absolutely clear that this is what they want, doctors and nurses are more likely to succeed in pressing for local arrangements to provide high quality palliative care for people dying at home.

The initiatives described in Chapter One were created by teams of doctors, nurses and other professionals. They have been taken up by the Government and are being encouraged throughout the NHS and Social Services. This is in response to the interest of an ageing generation. We have seen our parents die and some of our friends. We begin to realise that we too will die. Many of us would prefer to die at home or in a care home rather than being admitted to hospital.

129

Among these initiatives the Preferred Priorities for Care[20] has the specific aim of enabling a dying patient to choose their place of death and to receive the care which meets their individual needs and wishes.

THE ADVANCE DECISION AND THE PLACE OF DEATH

The hospital embodies a system for keeping people alive. That *is* what we want primarily of our hospitals. The NHS has been accused of systemic ageism and there have been calls to tackle ageism and promote equality in the NHS.[24] Because of this accusation doctors may be on the defensive, not wishing to appear ageist by suggesting that active life sustaining treatment be withheld.

The system has its own momentum, and a dying person, who should perhaps be allowed to die peacefully, gets carried along.

Many people who are frail and elderly , or terminally ill, retain mental capacity and can speak for themselves as death approaches. When a patient who is terminally ill has lost mental capacity an Advance Decision shows that in some circumstances, allowing the patient to die is acceptable, in fact what the patient would want. Care home staff, community nurses and GPs are very sensitive to patient's wishes to stay put and not be admitted to hospital. They appreciate the clarity of an Advance Decision and the outline of the patient's hopes, fears and wishes in a Statement of Values. With these they are very willing to discuss with the family, and come to an agreement about the care of the patient and the preferred place of death.

MY STATEMENT OF VALUES

This Statement of Values is attached to my Advance Decision.

To my family, doctors and nurses: Should I lose mental capacity, this is my statement of values, giving my wishes for my personal care, the background and motivation for my Advance Decision, what I want to happen to my body after death, and wishes for my funeral ceremony.

Signed..

Date..............................

Preferences for my daily care

These are my preferences only. Do what is feasible. The lives of other members of the family are more important than my life which is passing. Please meet their needs.

I would prefer:

To die at home – in my own home or that of a family member, or in a familiar care home.

To have my hair cut neatly, and my nails short. No nail varnish.

To wear my own clothes.

To wear spectacles, hearing aid and teeth (if I need them and can tolerate them.)   (Please clean and maintain them for me!).

To wash or be washed with cream soap and to have my skin moisturised.

Even if I am not mentally capable, I will enjoy:

Having a window opened and breathing the fresh air on a warm day,

Looking out of the window,

131

Watching the birds,

Listening to my own music,

Watching films (with another person preferably). I just

Like the colours, I don't expect to follow the plot!

Looking at my books of paintings and photographs.

I have always enjoyed food and drink. I like to drink from a china mug or a glass.

Please give me proper coffee (black), and very weak tea – Lapsang or Earl Grey, also without milk. I like fruit with yoghurt, fruit juice diluted with soda, fruit smoothies and ice-cream. If I refuse these, time to go!

Give me prunes! I do not want to get constipated. Please do not offer me milk or milky drinks or milk puddings.

I have given copies of my Advance Decision to Refuse life-sustaining Treatment to family members and to my GP and hospital consultant.

Background and motivation for my Advance Decision.
The background to my Advance Decision includes the deaths I have witnessed as a doctor as a daughter, and seeing the Advance Decision in action. The circumstances of my parents' deaths, my mother from Alzheimer's, and my father from stroke, persuaded me to write one now, while still in good health, and not to wait until I became ill.

My motivation to write an Advance Decision comes from a wish to face death realistically and stoically, a fear of losing my mind, and an unwillingness to die in indignity, being remembered that way by my family. I fear pain, and want my pain to be relieved, even if this appears to hasten my death. I fear artificial nutrition by nasogastric or PEG tube.

I want those around me to accept my death, to be kind, and to be spiritually aware. I know my family will care about me, and I trust them to carry out my wishes as far as possible. I hope someone I love will be there with me at the end.

I am indebted to the doctors and nurses and the other people who have contributed to my care during my life, and especially thank those who will care during these last days of my life.

Below I describe situations I would regard as intolerable. I would prefer to be allowed to die a natural death than to continue in such a situation:

Ongoing mental disability to the extent that I lack mental capacity and am unable to respond to the love of my family or the kindness of friends and helpers , and unable to find meaning and enjoyment in any activities. (I will be grateful for help with any activities, so long as I still have enough mental capacity to enjoy them)

Physical disability - weakness, breathlessness, lack of movement or coordination, sensory loss, or severe pain, to an extent that independent function is a struggle and I have become a burden to myself and others in even basic activities such as eating and drinking, reading or listening to books, going to the toilet, bathing, dressing, taking part in conversation.

Please see *What Choices Have I Made?* regarding what happens to my body after death, and my funeral. Note that I have registered with the NHS Organ Donation Registry.

REFERENCES

1. Kingsley Amis (1922-1995) *'Delivery Guaranteed'.*

2. *Review of the National Statistician of Deaths in England and Wales, 2008. Table 12: Place of death by age.* Office of National Statistics, 2010.

3. *End of Life Care Services.* The National Audit Office 26 November 2008. The Stationery Office: London.

4. *Healthy Life Expectancy.* Bulletin of the Parliamentary Office for Science and Technology No 257 - February 2006.

5. *Health Expectancies in the UK 2002.* Health Statistics Quarterly No 29. Office of National Statistics - 2006.

6. Newton P. *Personal View: A Good Death, but no thanks to the NHS.* British Medical Journal 2007; 334:536.

7. Duerden MG. *We need a mix of care in the NHS.* British Medical Journal. 2007; 334:599.

8. Health: Hospital acquired infections Column GC139 *Hansard* 17 July 2008.

9. *Figures on MRSA Bloodstream Infections.* The MRSA Surveillance System. Department of Health Publications and Statistics 2007.

10. *Changes to the Mandatory Healthcare Associated Infection Surveillance System for Clostridium Difficile.* Chief Medical Officer, Department of Health 2008.

11. *Hungry to Be Heard. The Scandal of Malnourished People in Hospital.* Age Concern August 2006.

12. *Improving End of Life Care.* Leading Edge Issue No.12. The NHS Confederation November 2005.

13. Harris D, Richard B, and Khana P. *Palliative care for the elderly – a need unmet.* Geriatric Medicine July. 2006.

14. Murray SA, Kendall M, Boyd K, and Sheik A *Illness trajectories and palliative care.* British Medical Journal 2005; 330:1007.

15. *Review of the National Statistician on deaths in England and Wales 2008. Cause of Death by Sex and Age Group.* Office for National Statistics 2010.

16. de Zulueta P. (2006) *Care of the Dying: A Case Study.* The New Generalist, No 14 – Winter.

17. Fisken R. *Personal View: Elder Abuse 21ˢᵗ Century Style.* British Medical Journal 2006; 332: 801.

18. *The NHS Strategy for End of Life Care.* Department of Health 2008.

19. Storey L, Pemberton C, Howard A, O'Donnell L. *Place of death: Hobson's choice or patient's choice?* Cancer Nursing Practice 2003; 2:4:33-38.

20. *Preferred Priorities for Care (PPC).* Lancashire and South Cumbria Cancer Services Network, National PPC Review Team. University of Cumbria and South Lancashire, December 2007.

21. *End of Life Care for Adults. Service Delivery, Quality and Staffing.* Nice Quality Standard [Q513] National Institute for Health and Care Excellence. Website nice. org.uk 2015

22. *Services we Monitor, Inspect and Regulate.* Care Quality Commission. Independent Regulator of Health and Social Care in England. Website cqc.org.uk 2015.

23. *NHS Organ Donor Register.* Website organdonation. nhs.uk Tel: 0300 123 23 23.

24. Singh I, Ayjar A, Bhat S. *Tackling ageism and promoting equality in health care.* British Journal of Hospital Medicine 2005; 66(10): 510-511.

Chapter 7

Decisions About Your Body After Death

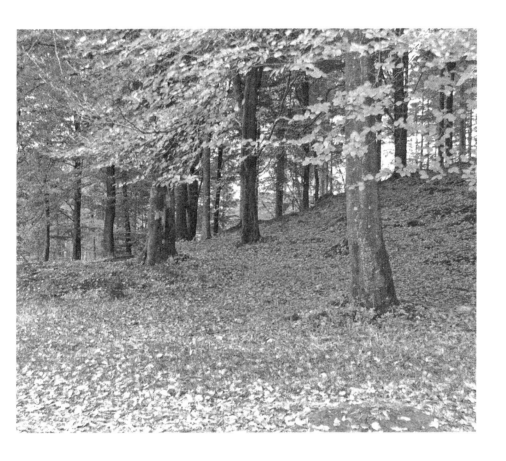

Then we shall 'ave ter bury thee!

*Members of Halifax Wesleyan Church on an outing
to the Cow and Calf Rocks, Ilkley Moor (1805).*

What happens to your body after death can affect the experience and grieving of your family. They may be too stunned or exhausted to think properly about what you would have wanted, or to think about what might comfort them. It will help if you make some plans.

There are many choices you can make in advance to help your family. They will be asked what should happen to your body immediately after your death. Organs or tissues can be donated for transplant. They may be asked to consent to a post-mortem. Your family will want to know what sort of funeral you would want and what your choice would be for cremation or burial. These and other choices are considered in this chapter.

Who Do You Want to Tend Your Body?

Soon after death, the body is washed, the eyes and mouth are closed, and the orifices blocked with cotton wool. Usually this is done by the nursing staff of the hospital or care home, or by the undertakers. You may prefer this idea of 'kind strangers' attending to your body after death, but in some cultures it is the norm for family members to wash and wrap the corpse.

Some people find it comforting that their family will tend their body after death, and some families are helped in their grief by doing this. Most hospitals, hospices and care homes will ensure privacy in a suitable room, and assist , if this is what they want, or this can be done in your own home if you have died there.

If you have died in hospital your body will be taken to the hospital mortuary and put in cold store, until it is collected by the funeral director, or by your family. It can be removed from there only in a suitable coffin and in a vehicle in which the coffin can be laid flat.

Where Do You Want Your Body Kept?

The funeral directors will have a variety of coffins to choose from. As well as traditional wood chip and veneer, or solid wood, there are environmentally friendly coffins or flamboyant personalised coffins. Alternatively, you can obtain the coffin yourself through one of many websites (just search for 'coffin') or you can make your own – full instructions are to be found in the *Natural Death Handbook*.[2]

The funeral directors will collect the body from the hospital mortuary or from the care home or your own home, and take it to their own chilled chapel of rest or quiet room. The funeral directors can simply wrap the body and place it in the coffin ready for the funeral or they can dress it in clothes which the family provide, leaving the face and hands uncovered, and place it in the uncovered coffin. The body can then be viewed in the funeral director's chapel or brought to your home the day before the funeral if that is what your family want.

People are generally unsure about seeing the body after death, but I found it helpful when my father died. Viewing the body is another stage in confronting death, talking or thinking about the one who has died, and saying goodbye.

PLAN YOUR FUNERAL

Funeral Directors

You might think that if your family use a funeral director they will be taken over, put into a production line, and end up with a rather impersonal funeral. In fact, funeral directors have changed with the times and are generally open to ideas and are as flexible as possible in trying to provide what is wanted. They know the crematoria and burial grounds in the locality and the staff who work there. They can negotiate personalised arrangements and will also take over most of the form filling and bureaucracy required for the funeral ceremony and disposal of the body.

139

There are two national associations through which you can find a funeral director[3,4] or you could ask around for local recommendations. You do not have to use a funeral director. Some people do everything themselves. Staff at the hospital, and at the crematorium or cemetery will give advice and provide the paperwork for certification of disposal of the body.

Funeral Ceremonies

For many people their religion will provide the form and structure for their funeral ceremony – usually at the place of worship of the deceased during life, and conducted by the religious leader who knew them.

But within the laws on Public Health and Environmental Protection and Nuisance there is great scope. It can be a great solace to plan a unique ceremony, indoors or outdoors, with singing, music, displays of photographs or objects, and the joint preparation of a funeral meal. The mourners can carry the coffin, light candles, reminisce, and read poetry.

The importance of the ceremony and disposal is the opportunity it provides for families and people who knew you to come to terms with death – your death, the deaths of other loved ones, and their own death. There is a healthy move to bring families into the planning and the ceremony itself, rather than just being passive consumers of a service. Some funeral directors are more in tune with this change than others.

Lack of involvement can be a cause for regret later. Up to half of mourners are said to be disappointed with the funeral ceremonies put together for their loved ones.[5] This is why discussing and writing down ideas for your own funeral or memorial service can be helpful to your family. They know they are doing what you would want. You can go further and purchase a policy with a local funeral director and leave instructions with them.[6] You should discuss this with your family first to avoid them feeling hurt that you have not involved them sufficiently.

CREMATION OR BURIAL? -And Other Options

Cremation

The most usual method of disposal is cremation. This can only be done in a crematorium. Noxious fumes may be generated as the body burns – for example from mercury fillings in the teeth - and there are public health problems from an incompletely cremated body. Therefore, your body cannot be cremated on the beach or in your garden. The crematorium is managed to ensure complete cremation with minimal emissions, which are monitored.

The crematorium is a bland environment because it is nondenominational; though in the United Kingdom it most closely resembles a church. There are facilities for recorded music to be played, and often an organ or piano. Any ceremony that you wish can be performed, or none, for there is no law requiring a ceremony. A member of your family, a friend, or your own religious leader can preside, or the crematorium can provide a chaplain or other religious leader. The ceremony does not need to represent any system of belief. It can simply be made up of music, reminiscences and readings, and whatever you want to include.

Your ashes from cremation may be scattered anywhere: in the crematorium grounds, in your garden, in the countryside or at sea, or kept in an urn, or buried. The only restriction is that if buried in a container, ashes must not be moved without a licence from the Home Office.[7] This is pertinent if they are buried in your garden and later your family wish to move house. Your family must declare the burial site to the new occupier, to avoid their distress should they find the urn while gardening.

Burial

The other common method of disposal is burial, traditionally in a churchyard (presumably after a religious ceremony and

141

committal), or local cemetery. It is possible to book your place and perhaps pay for it in advance. Churchyards may be short of space and be willing to accept only regular worshippers at the church or those who have a parent or spouse already buried there. Local Authority cemeteries must always find a space, but possibly not exactly where you would like.

Most cemeteries now offer only what are known as lawn graves —a simple small headstone with grass which can be mown in contiguity with the rest of the graves in the cemetery, like a lawn. It is unlikely you will be allowed a tall headstone because they can become unstable, and therefore dangerous.

Woodland or meadow burial grounds are relatively new. There is likely to be one reasonably close. These have a beneficial impact on the environment and provide great freedom as to the choice of ceremony.

Liquefaction; Freeze Drying

These are developments for the future motivated by the need to reduce the impact on the environment. These processes produce less smoke and toxins than cremation and take up less space than burial. The body is rendered to a small amount of material suitable to return to the earth.

Disposal of your Body at Sea

This is expensive and complicated -not something to be embarked upon as a whim. It requires permission from the Marine and Fisheries Agency[8] (to protect the sea and the fish) and from the coroner (to protect us from foul play. Once buried at sea, a corpse cannot be recovered for further examination.) There can be problems with burial at sea; a corpse can be washed ashore or taken up in fishing gear, causing distress. Having your ashes scattered at sea after cremation is a less complicated alternative.

142

Burial on Your Own Land (field, wood or garden)

This is permissible so long as there is no possibility of fouling a water course. The local environmental health department or water company would have an interest. A funeral director would make enquiries for you. The site must be registered. If the land is sold the purchaser can require your family to seek Home Office permission and to pay to have the remains removed.

POST-MORTEM EXAMINATION

A post-mortem may be demanded by the coroner, or requested by the doctor. It may be traumatic for your family to be asked about post-mortem. You can help them in this eventuality by thinking about it now and deciding what your own attitude and wishes would be.

Post-mortem Requested by the Coroner

The role of the coroner is to confirm that death occurred from natural causes, or to detect foul play, self-harm, neglect or negligence. The Coroner's request for a post-mortem cannot be refused, even by those whose religion precludes post-mortem. The coroner might agree to a post mortem by medical imaging in exceptional circumstances. In the case of a person dying of old age or terminal illness, known to their doctor, referral to the coroner would be unusual. A post-mortem will be requested if no doctor has seen the deceased in the 14 days before death.

Post-mortem Requested by the Doctor

A post-mortem might be requested by the doctors who had been looking after a patient, to gain a more complete understanding of the illness which caused death. Aspects of an illness are sometimes confirmed at post-mortem which were not apparent when the patient was alive. It would be surprising if there were not occasionally something more to learn by a detailed post-mortem examination. In this way the post-mortem also contributes to good practice, medical education and research.

143

In a full post-mortem all the organs are examined, in a partial post-mortem only those organs involved in the fatal disease are examined. Blocks or fragments of tissue may be retained for research or for future examination as new diagnostic or genetic tests become available, or for medical education.

After the post-mortem, your family will receive an outline report (or a more detailed report if they request it) including information about tissues which have been retained.

Consent for a Post-mortem
In seeking consent to a post-mortem the doctor must give the family full information which will include asking permission to retain tissues.[9] Your family must be asked to consent, therefore a statement in your living will would help them to decide about it. If you write a Statement of Values you can express your willingness for a post-mortem, that you agree to retention of tissues or organs, and that the hospital should dispose of these remains with dignity. Alternatively, you can state that you prefer there to be no post-mortem.

THE NHS ORGAN DONOR REGISTER [10]
If you decide you would like to donate organs or tissue after your death, you can register with the NHS Organ Donor Register, which ensures organs and tissues are harvested and made available to recipients who need them. Driving licences issued since 1993 have a box to tick if you want to be on the organ donor register.

Through feedback from donors' families, and recipients, the UK Transplant Organisation is aware of the gratitude of recipients and the comfort to bereaved families. Grieving families find it difficult to consent to organs or tissue being taken, but later gain comfort and hope from knowing that they have done what you wanted and that some good has come from your death.

In old age, or after a long terminal illness, organs and tissues may not be suitable for donation. After the age of 75 years, only the cornea can be donated.

Human Immune Deficiency Virus (HIV) and some other rare infections, and some treatments, for example recent treatment with radioactive isotopes would preclude donation.

The current situation in the UK is that donors have to opt in by registering. A family cannot offer the organs of an adult who is not registered, (although currently they can refuse after you are dead even if you have registered). You can register online or obtain a registration form at your GP's surgery or the local pharmacy. When you register you receive a donor card to carry around with you or keep at home. Tell your family that you have registered.

Organ Donation
Organ donation is the donation for transplant of a whole organ. The kidneys, heart, lung, liver and pancreas can be donated. Only a small proportion of people die in circumstances where they are able to donate their organs. Since organs have to be harvested soon after someone has died, they can only be retrieved from a person who has died in hospital. Usually organs come from people who are certified dead while on a ventilator in a hospital intensive care unit generally as a result of brain haemorrhage, a major accident (such as a car crash), or a stroke.

Tests are done to ensure that all signs of life have gone in the brain stem, which maintains the heartbeat and respiration (see Chapter Two), and that all other brain activity has also ceased. These tests are done by two doctors (one a consultant), who are not connected with the team of doctors looking after you, or with the transplant team.

The purpose of continuing ventilation after death is only to maintain the oxygen supply to the organs so that they will be viable for the recipient.

In my Statement of Values *I have made it clear that should my organs be suitable for transplant I accept ventilation after my death, until my organs can be harvested.*

Tissue Donation

Other parts of the body can be donated not as whole organs but as parts of organs or tissues. These include skin, bone, joints, blood vessels, heart valves and the cornea of the eye. Tissues remain viable for donation for some time after death, and ventilation is not required.

DONATING THE BRAIN FOR RESEARCH

The Parkinson's Disease Society[11] maintains a tissue bank of both normal and abnormal brain tissue from brains donated after death. Tissue is provided after careful evaluation of their research proposals to researchers who are looking for a cure for Parkinson's disease and other brain diseases.

DONATION OF YOUR BODY

Medical students learn anatomy by the dissection of a human body. They are usually taught by junior doctors who are training to be surgeons and who themselves must gain a deeper and more thorough knowledge of anatomy. Anatomy is also part of the training of dentists, nurses and physiotherapists.

It is the duty of the Medical School to ensure that students behave with decorum and respect in the dissecting room and that no tissue is removed from there. Most students are awed and humbled by the privilege of being able to see what is normally hidden beneath the skin. They are amazed at the intricacies and brought down to earth by the realities of the body. Shared humanity is acknowledged.

Should you decide to donate your body the Human Tissue Authority[12] will put you in touch with a medical school. Forms need to be completed well in advance and enacted as soon as death occurs. At the end of dissection the body is placed in a coffin for burial or cremation after a simple funeral paid for by the medical school. If the relatives wish, they can appoint a funeral director to collect the coffin and organise the ceremony themselves.

WHAT CHOICES HAVE I MADE?

These are the choices I have made for my body after death. This document is part of my Statement of Values attached to my Advance Decision.

I am content for my body after death to be tended by whoever has been looking after me - nurses, care home staff or members of my family.

I would like to be dressed so that members of my family may view my body after death if they wish to.

My funeral ceremony should last about an hour, with music and poetry chosen by my family to remind them of me.

Afterwards, have a good party with nice food and music.

I want my body to be cremated and my ashes placed, not scattered, under the heather by a rock in a place members of the family love.

If the doctors request a post-mortem, please consent.

I have registered with the NHS organ donor register. Please let the doctors know, and give consent if donation is requested. I accept ventilation after my death should any of my organs be suitable for transplant.

Please donate my brain to the Parkinson's Disease Society, with whom I have registered.

REFERENCES

1. Anon: Thought to be members of Halifax Wesleyan Church on a visit to the Cow and Calf Rocks, Ilkley. *"On Ilkley Moor 'baht 'at"*. Tune 'Cranbrook' (1805) Thomas Clarke.

2. Eds: Wienrich S, Speyer J. *The Natural Death Handbook*. The Natural Death Centre, Winchester 2003.Web site: naturaldeath.org.uk.

3. *National Association of Funeral Directors*, 618 Warwick Road, Solihull, West Midlands, B91 1AA. Tel: 0845 230 1343. Website: nafd.org.uk.

4. *Society of Allied and Independent Funeral Directors*, 3 Bullfields, Sawbridgeworth, Herts CM2 9DB. Tel: 0845 2306777.Website: saif.org.uk.

5. *Minerva*. British Medical Journal 2005; 330: 428.

6. Paul Harris. *What to do when someone dies*. Which. London 2005. Web site: Which.co.uk.

7. North Tyneside Local Authority.2009. Web site: northtyneside.gov.uk.

8. *Burial at Sea of Human Remains*. Marine Fisheries Agency. Department for the Environment, Food and Rural Affairs 2009. Web site: mfa.gov.uk/environment/works/burial

9. *Human Tissue Act 2004*. Office of Public Sector Information. Web site: opsi.gov.uk.

10. *NHS Organ Donor Register*. UK Transplant Service. Tel: 0300 123 23 23 open 24 hrs. Web site: uktransplantservice.org.uk.

11. *UK Parkinson's Disease Society Tissue Bank.* Imperial College, 160 DuCane Road, London W12 0NN. Website: parkinsons.org.uk.

12. *Human Tissue Authority.* Finlayson House 15-17 Furnival Street, London EC4 1AB. Tel: 0207 269 1900. Website: hta.gov.uk.

Chapter 8

What Shall I Do Now?

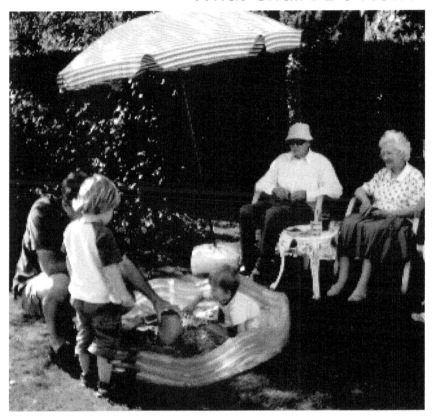

"Oh, oh, oh!" she cried
as the ambulance men lifted her to the stretcher -
"Is this what you call
making me comfortable?"

William Carlos Williams (1883-1963)
The Last Words of My English Grandmother

SO WHAT SHOULD I DO NOW?

1.Write an Advance Decision and talk about it with your family.
Write an Advance Decision, in case at some time in the future you lose mental capacity. If you become terminally ill and need medical treatment, doctors will assess your mental capacity and discuss the Advance Decision with your family or representative, before acting on it.

Discuss your Advance Decision with your family or the people you want doctors to talk to about your medical treatment should you lose mental capacity. Give copies to your family, your GP and also your hospital consultant.

You do not need the input of a doctor or a lawyer to write an Advance Decision.

My advice is not to make detailed instructions, but if you have a progressive disease, you may (if you wish) specify in detailed instructions the treatment which you refuse and the clinical circumstances in which this should apply. Discuss detailed instructions with your doctor.

2. Write a Statement of Values.
Outline the background and motivation for your Advance Decision, and describe the situations in which you would not wish to go on living, should you lose mental capacity. Discuss with your family, so that they will know what your wishes would be regarding life sustaining treatment. Say where you would wish to die and outline aspects of your personal care which would be important to you. You may refer to your wish for a DNAR agreement in certain circumstances.

Mention your Organ Donor Registration and include your wishes for your funeral ceremony and burial or cremation of your body.

You can also say what you think about assisted suicide and euthanasia. This is illegal now, but the law might could change in future.

3. Register with the NHS Organ Donor Registry.

4. For financial affairs – grant the Power of Attorney.
Appoint someone to have the Lasting Power of Attorney to handle your *financial affairs*, should you become mentally incapable. (If you have already made an Enduring Power of Attorney, this still stands). *However there are few circumstances in which you should appoint a welfare attorney.*

5. Think about a 'Do Not Attempt to Resuscitate' (DNAR) agreement.
At some point in future, if you become very ill, you (or those close to you) might wish to make a 'Do Not Attempt to Resuscitate' (DNAR) agreement. Those people looking after you at the time, will then know not to attempt resuscitation if a cardiac or respiratory arrest occurs.

6. If you hope to die at home, plan in advance.
Seeing out the end of your days at home requires Advance Planning with your community nursing team and your General Practitioner. If your needs can be met quickly in a crisis, there is more likelihood of avoiding emergency hospital admission against your wishes.

7. If, when you are frail and ill, an operation is proposed, ask questions.
When someone is very frail and ill, it is a difficult decision whether to operate or not. Ask questions about the risks and likely benefit, and whether there are any alternatives to operation If you lose mental capacity your Advance Decision and Statement of Values are a guide to your wishes, which may suggest that palliative care might be more appropriate than an operation.

8. Help your family to plan after your death.
You can do this by thinking about some of the choices which have to be made and giving guidance in your statement of values. Choices include the response to a request for post-mortem examination, organ or tissue donation, funeral arrangements and the method of disposal of your body.

THE MOST IMPORTANT STEP IS:

Write an Advance Decision and talk about it with your family
Read from page 57-65 and see my own Advance Decision on page 74-80. The form on page xx provides a possible template for you. The form can also be found at my website: advancedecision.uk

SUMMARY: WHAT SHALL I DO NOW?

1. Write an Advance Decision and talk about it with your

family.

2. Write a Statement of Values.

3. Register with the NHS Organ Donor Registry.

4. For financial affairs – grant the Power of Attorney.

5. Think about a 'Do Not Attempt to Resuscitate' (DNAR)

agreement.

6. If you want to die at home, plan in advance.

7. If, when you are very frail or ill, an operation is proposed,

ask questions.

8. Help your family by making plans for after your death.

Appendix

Living Will Form

Please cut out or copy, and use this form as a template for your Advance Decision.

The form may also be obtained at website *www.advancedecision.co.uk.*

On the form, italics are used for the basic content, referenced in Ch. 4. Spaces for your personal details and instructions which you may write in your own words are headed in a different font and the spaces left blank.

In my Advance Decision (pp 72-80) I have written my own words in these spaces. You may copy them, but they become your own words.

As the author of this book I cannot be held responsible for anything written by the reader or any action taken or not taken by a medical practitioner.

Living Will

ADVANCE DECISION
of

....

Date....................

Taken from:

What Shall I Do About My Death
Published November 2015
www.advancedecision.uk

Advance Decision to Refuse Treatment

To my family, my doctors and everyone concerned: this Decision is made by me when I am of sound mind, well informed and after careful consideration. If in future I lose mental capacity, and am terminally ill, in the clinical circumstances described I refuse life sustaining treatment, even though my life will be at risk and my death may be hastened as a result.

My Name	Any distinguishing features in the event of unconsciousness
Address	Date of Birth
	Telephone Number(s)

Mental Capacity

Please do not assume I have lost capacity. Find out about my medical history from my family, GP or hospital notes. I might need help and time to communicate.

Legal status

If I have lost mental capacity please check the validity and applicability of this Advance Decision. It must be taken into account in decisions about my medical care. I have indicated clinical circumstances when, if I am terminally ill and have lost mental capacity, I refuse life sustaining treatment. This does not preclude basic care and comfort.

Statement of Values

Please read my Statement of Values which outlines the background and motivation for my Advance Decision. It indicates clinical situations which I would find intolerable. Talk to my family, to help consider whether I would wish to refuse life sustaining treatment.

Applicable clinical circumstances

Loss of Mental Capacity

I have become unable to participate effectively in decisions about my medical care through loss of mental capacity or unconsciousness and

Two independent doctors (one a consultant) are of the opinion that I am unlikely to recover from illness or impairment and

Terminal Illness

I suffer from one or more of the following:

Advanced Alzheimer's disease or any other form of dementia;

Severe and lasting brain damage due to injury, stroke, disease or other cause;

Advanced degenerative disease of the nervous system (e.g. motor neurone disease);

Severe immune deficiency (e.g. AIDS);

Advanced cancer with secondary dissemination not responsive to treatment;

Severe and increasing disability from terminal cardiac or respiratory disease;

Any other condition of comparable gravity.

*(Schedule taken from Notes for Guidance to NHS staff when assessing an Advance Decision)

My Decision

In the clinical circumstances described above,

I refuse any medical intervention or treatment aimed solely at prolonging or sustaining my life, even though my life may be at risk as a result.

If my Advance Decision should take effect, please institute a Do Not Attempt to Resuscitate (DNAR) agreement.

Any distressing symptoms (including any caused by lack of food) are to be fully controlled by appropriate analgesia or other treatment, even though that treatment may shorten my life.

Unconsciousness due to brain damage

Pregnancy (Applicable / Non-Applicable)
If I am pregnant and suffering from any of the clinical circumstances described above I wish to receive medical treatment or procedures to sustain my life in the hope of safe delivery of my child. Once my child is delivered I wish to reinstate my wishes as set out in this document.

Organ Donation (Applicable / Non-Applicable)
I have registered with the NHS Organ Donor register. After brain death I wish for life support necessary to maintain for a time the viability of any of my organs or tissues suitable for donation.

My Advance Decision to refuse life prolonging treatment is to be followed even if my life is at risk as a result.

My Signature   **Date of Signature**

Witness Statement

The maker of this Decision signed it in my presence. I do not know of any pressure brought on him/her to make such a Decision and I believe it was made by his/her own wish. I do not stand to gain from his/her death.

Witness	Signed
Name	Telephone Number(s)
Address	Date
Witness	Signed
Name	Telephone Number(s)
Address	Date

My General Practitioner is: (Name)
Address
Telephone
The name of my Welfare Attorney is: (applicable / non-applicable)

The following list identifies people who have a copy and with whom I have discussed this Advance Decision to Refuse Treatment. Their contact details are provided. Any of them may be informed in a situation where I require medical care but have lost mental capacity to take part in discussions and decisions about treatment.

Name	Relationship	Telephone Number

Statement of Values (Recommended)

Here you should attach a Statement of Values in your own words, or a letter to your family.

Detailed Instructions
(Optional - delete as required below)

Applicable

See detailed instructions below.

Non-Applicable

This Advance Decision was made **without** detailed instructions.

Index

A

Advance Decision 52-78, 2-5, 12, 14, 34, 160.

applicable clinical circumstances 38, 45, 59, 65, 76 .

and choosing where to die 74, 103, 106, 130.

how to write 64-80, 75.

and life sustaining treatment 36-37, 41-44, 46-49, 64, 75.

and resuscitation 63, 87-88.

Advance Directive 3, 52.

Advance Planning 108, 120, 125-130, 153.

Age

and choosing where to die 94-96, 106-107.

and dying 14-15, 30, 112-113.

and life sustaining operations 49-51.

Advance Statement see Statement of Values.

Age UK 2, 14-15, 30, 81,87.

Alzheimer's disease 20, 71, 81, 82-83.

See also Dementia.

Alzheimer's Society 71.

Admission to hospital 7, 23, 26, 107, 114-116, 126..

See also Life-sustaining treatment, Medical emergencies.

Anaesthetic 42, 45, 47, 51.

Aneurysm, aortic 17, 50.

Angina 21, 23.

Antibiotics 43, 85.

Artificial hydration 19-20, 29, 37-42, 84-85.

Artificial nutrition 19-20, 24, 37-40, 105, 106.

Assessment of Mental Capacity. See Mental Capacity.

Assisted Dying 8, 65, 128.

Attorney. See Lasting Power of Attorney.

Audit Commission. See *National Audit Office.*

B

Bedsore (pressure ulcer) 25, 29.

Bill on Assisted Dying for the Terminally Ill 8.

Blood pressure 22, 51.

Blood transfusion 43.

Brain 16, 24-25, 48, 60, 67, 72, 103, 146.

   See also Stroke.

Brain stem 16, 17, 28.

Breathing 16, 22, 45, 47, 146.

   See also Respiratory support, Ventilation.

Breathlessness 23-24, 27, 33, 45. 102.

Burial 141-142.

C

Cancer 7-8, 14-15, 40, 87, 117.

   and Advance Decisions 36, 67, 87.

   trajectory of 28, 118.

Capacity. See Mental Capacity.

Cardiac defibrillation 84.

Cardiopulmonary resuscitation (CPR) 4, 84-85, 102-103.

   See also Do Not Attempt to Resuscitate.

Care home 7, 14, 29, 108, 113.

   See also Nursing home, Residential home

Care. See Palliative; Personal; Statement of Values

Care Quality Commission 7-8, 127.

Cause of Death 14-30, 117-125.

Cerebrovascular disease. See Stroke.

Chemotherapy 26, 54.

Chest infection 16, 22, 28.

Chest pain. See Angina.

Choice

    of place of death 7, 14, 108, 117-131.

    your body after death 138-147.

Chronic disease 21-23, 113.

Circulation 14-16, 18, 43.

Clinical circumstances 36, 68-69, 74, 76-77, 89, 91.

Clostridium Difficile 118.

Coffin 138-139.

Communication, difficulties with 40,61.

    See also Family, doctors and nurses communicating with.

Community 6-7, 18, 24, 27.

Community nursing 7, 108, 120-122, 126-130.

Compassion in Dying 71, 81.

Competence. See Mental Capacity.

Consciousness 21, 40-41, 46-49, 102.

    See also Unconsciousness, Persistent vegetative state.

Consent

    for operation 40, 51.

    for post-mortem 144.

    to medical treatment 62.

Coronary artery disease 21.

    See also Heart disease.

Coroner 143-144.

Court of Protection 64, 65, 69, 89, 95.

Cremation 120, 123.

D

Death 2, 33, 127.

See also Cause of death and Place of death.

Decision. See Advance Decision.

Defibrillation, cardiac 102.

See also Do Not Attempt to Resuscitate,

Cardiopulmonary resuscitation.

Dehydration 18, 19, 35-36.

Dementia 14-15, 20, 28.

and artificial nutrition 20, 40.

and Advance Decision 62, 69, 82.

trajectory of and place of death 28, 105.

Detailed Instructions 80, 83, 88-92, 152.

Diabetes 22.

Dialysis, renal 44.

Disability 26, 66-68, 79, 100.

learning disability 60-61.

due to long standing illness 113.

Disposal of body138-147.

District nurse. See Community nurse.

Do Not Attempt to Resuscitate (DNAR) 4, 36, 59, 84. 86, 90, 102-108.

Cardiopulmonary resuscitation.

See also Resuscitation.

Doctors and nurses. Communication. See Family

Donation of body 146.

   of brain 146.

   See also Organ donation.

Dying 14-17, 21-33, 112, 117, 125-130.

E

Emergency. See Medical emergency.

End of Life Care. See Advance planning, NHS strategy, NICE guidance for, Palliative care, Terminal care.

Endotracheal tube 46.

   See also Tracheostomy.

F

Family or representative 65, 125, 129, 131-133, 138, 152, 154.

   See also Applicable clinical circumstances,

   Detailed instructions, Head injury, Statement of Values,

   Welfare attorney.

Forms

   for disposal of body 139.

   for Advance Decision 73-80, 81, 82, Appendix,

   advancedecision.uk.

   for organ donation 148.

Funerals, Funeral Directors 139-141.

G

General Medical Council 34, 57-58, 88.

General Practitioner (GP). 8, 77, 126, 130.

   See also Family.

Gold Standards Framework 6.

H

Head injury 41, 47.

See also Unconsciousness, Persistent unconsciousness.

Headway 86.

Heart attack 17, 22-23, 36, 84-85, 102.

Heart disease 14-15, 21, 30, 86.

    trajectory of 23-24, 119.

Heartbeat 14-15, 17, 24, 43, 84-85.

HIV 69, 145.

Home, own 6-7, 27, 108, 112-3, 120, 122, 129.

    See also Care home, Nursing home, Residential home.

Hospice 15, 112, 117.

Hospital 5, 15, 39, 114-117, 120-121.

    admission to 24, 26, 91, 121, 125.

    acquired infection 116.

    nutrition 116.

    See also Emergencies.

How to:

    appoint an Attorney (LPA) 94.

    engage with Advance Planning 125-130.

    prevent hospital admission 108, 125-130.

    register for organ donation 144.

    write an Advance Decision 64-80.

    write a statement of Values 131-133.

I

Incapacity. See Mental Capacity, loss of.

Infection 20, 41.

    chest infection, 16, 22-24.

    hospital acquired infection 116.

K

Kidney 17, 38, 44.

L

Lasting Power of Attorney (LPA).

  personal welfare 93-96.

  property and affairs 92.

Legal standing of an Advance Decision 58, 73, 75, 82, 88.

Life sustaining treatment 38-51, 111, 149, 106, 130.

  and Advance Decision 36-37, 41-44, 46-49, 70.

Liverpool Primary Care Pathway 7.

Living Will. See Advance Decision, Statement of Values.

Local Authority. See Social Services.

Loss of appetite 19-20.

Lungs 22-23.

  See also Pulmonary embolism, respiratory disease.

M

MacMillan Cancer Support 119.

Marie Curie Cancer Care 8, 119.

Medic Alert 66.

Medical emergencies 7, 24, 36-37, 103.

  and Advance Decision 36, 45, 57, 59.

  and resuscitation 36, 45, 103, 84, 90.

  and choice of where to die 108, 120-123.

Memory, loss of. See Mental capacity, Dementia.

Mental capacity

  definition 60.

  loss of 25-26, 67, 73.

assessment 63-64.

possibly restored 47-48.

retained 59.

Mental Capacity Act 4, 60, 70, 92.

Morphine 32-33.

Motor Neurone Disease 45,46, 66, 83, 84.

Motor Neurone Disease Association 81, 84.

Multiple Resistant Staphylococcus Aureus (MRSA)116.

Multiple Sclerosis 64, 83, 85.

Multiple Sclerosis Society 81, 85.

N

National Audit Office 5, 15, 107, 117.

National Confidential Enquiry into Patient Outcomes and Death (NCEPOD) 49-51.

National Confidential Enquiry into Post Operative Deaths (NCEPOD) 49.

National Health Service (NHS) 116, 118, 126, 129.

End of Life Care Strategy 6, 125, 129.

Organ Donor Register 126, 160.

National Institute for Health and Clinical Excellence (NICE) Guidance for End of Life Care. 7-8, 127.

Natural death 9.

Neurodegenerative disease 46, 64, 69, 83.

Nursing care 18, 24, 27-29, 37-38, 39.

community nursing 7, 108, 113.

Nursing home 24, 27, 112, 113, 123.

Nutrition, artificial 19-21, 26, 27, 39-42, 124.

O

Office of the Public Guardian 93-96.

Old age 15, 30, 124.

Operations 39, 49-51, 153.

consent for 40, 51.

deaths after 449-51.

for cancer 19.

of benefit in elderly 50.

Organ donation 128, 144, 153.

Organ failure 18, 30.

See also brain, heart, kidney, liver, lung.

P

Pacemaker 42.

Pain 28, 31.

Palliative care 31, 49, 51, 92, 117.

Parkinson's Association 81, 85, 146.

Parkinson's Disease 63, 85.

Patients' Association 81, 87.

Percutaneous endogastric (PEG) tube 39.

See also Artificial nutrition.

Peritoneal dialysis 44.

See also Renal dialysis.

Persistent Vegetative State 48, 49

Personal care 28, 52, 106, 108-109, 111, 132.

Place of death 2, 15, 108, 112-130.

Post operative deaths49-51. See also *NCEPOD*.

Post-mortem 143-144.

Preferred Place of Death 2, See also Place of death.

Preferred Priorities for Care 7, See also Advance Planning, Personal care.

Pressure ulcer 25, 29.

Public Guardian. See Office of, Court of Protection.

Pulmonary embolism 17, 25, 116.

Q

Quality of care See *Care Quality Commission.*

R

Radiotherapy 36, 54.

Residential home 113. See also Care home

Respiratory disease 14-15, 22-24, 45-47.

  trajectory of 22-23, 102.

  See also Breathing, Chest infection.

Respiratory support 45-47, 84.

Resuscitation 24.

  and Advance Decision 63, 87-88, 104, 106.

  and life-sustaining treatment 36, 46.

  See also Do Not Attempt to Resuscitate (DNAR).

S

Sedation 33, 46.

Social Services 5, 127, 129. See also Care home.

Speech 26, 37, 40.

Speech and Language Therapist (SALT) 37.

Statement of Values 56, 63, 67, 78-79, 91, 128, 131-133, 147, 152.

Stroke 15, 24, 69.

  and artificial nutrition 42.

trajectory of 25-26, 121.

Stroke Association 26, 34.

Sudden death 17, 25, 102.

T

Terminal care 30-33, 106. See also End of life care,
Palliative care.

Terminal illness 14, 17, 29, 68-69, 74.

Thirst 18, 38.

Thrombosis, deep vein. 17, 25.

Tracheostomy (tracheotomy) 48.

Trajectory of disease 21, 23-25, 28-29, 117-124.

Transient ischemic attack (TIA) 24.

Transplant 75, 120, 144-146.

U

Unconsciousness 39, 41, 46, 47, 71, 72, 102. See also Persistent
unconsciousness.

V

Validity of Advance Decision 54, 58-59, 160.

Ventilation 45-47, 49, 83-84. See also Respiratory support.

W

Welfare attorney 77, 93-96. See also Lasting Power of Attorney.

Witnesses 65, 67, 76, 95, 136.

Lightning Source UK Ltd.
Milton Keynes UK
UKOW05f1227231016

285944UK00005B/24/P